A to Z of Good Sex

A to Z of Good Sex

Dr David Delvin

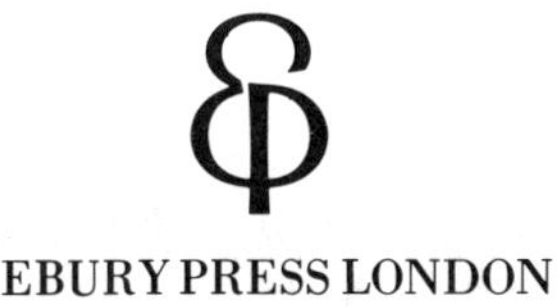

EBURY PRESS LONDON

PUBLISHED BY EBURY PRESS
an imprint of Century Hutchinson Ltd
Brookmount House
62–65 Chandos Place
London WC2 4NW

British Library Cataloguing in Publication Data.
Delvin, David
A–Z of Good Sex: Your Questions Answered
1. Sex relations
I. title
306.7

ISBN 0–85223–768–5

Editor Viv Croot
Designed by Adrian Morris Publishing Ltd
Cover photograph Norman Mosaliem
Transworld Features

Computerset by Chapterhouse, The Cloisters, Formby L37 3PX
Printed and bound in Great Britain at The Bath Press, Avon

FOREWORD

Q My husband likes to pour a little of his favourite 1977 Burgundy over my body before we make love. Is there anything wrong with this, doctor?

A There is indeed, ma'am! I know that society is still pretty permissive these days, but there are certain standards which have to be maintained, aren't there?

The correct year would be '73 or a '70 – or even (dare I say it) a '69 . . . .

That question and answer, dear reader, will give you some insight into the slightly dotty 'Love, Sex and Health' column which I've been writing for that splendid women's magazine SHE over the last 17 years. This book is mainly based on that column.

I'd like to pay tribute to its successive Editors – and, in particular, to its current Editor-in-Chief, the dynamic and glamorous Joyce Hopkirk – for letting me speak totally frankly and honestly in my answers to people's sexual questions. No other woman's magazine has ever been so unembarrassed and uninhibited about what it prints.

I hope that our selection of material will not only help you to make your sex life safer and more fun, but also bring a chuckle to your lips. For laughter in bed is, after all, a precious commodity – more valuable than 1,000 orgasms. (Mind you, 1,000 orgasms aren't bad either.)

Dr. David Delvin

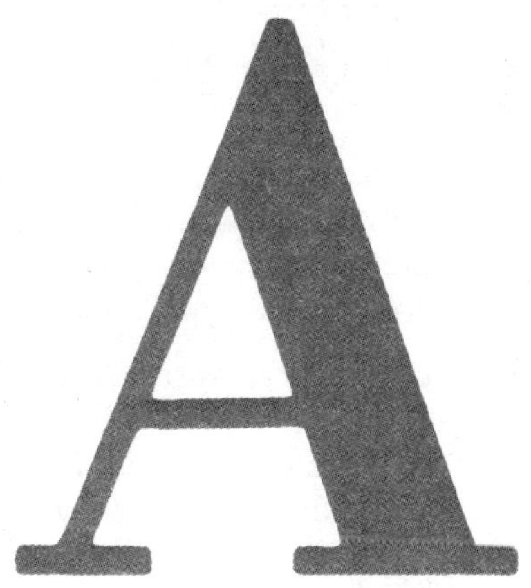

Adultery

'Infants', as somebody once remarked, 'don't have nearly so much fun in infancy as adults do in adultery.' And that's the trouble with adultery. It's awfully tempting – and it always looks as though it would be such fun, and wouldn't do any real harm, would it?

Unfortunately, the trouble is that adultery quite often *does* do harm – to marriages and families, and to people's physical and emotional health.

Of course, it may well lead to divorce. Even today (when adultery is rather less frowned on than it was) about a third of all divorce petitions are brought on grounds of infidelity. In my opinion, the infidelity is usually the *symptom* of problems in marriage rather than their cause.

But there's no doubt that in most cases, if an innocent party finds out about his or her partner's adultery, this is likely to lead to a great deal of emotional upheaval – and sometimes even to violence. The trouble and bitterness may spill over and affect the children of the marriage, something no one in their right mind would want.

You must also bear in mind a couple of simple basic medical

facts, which are so often forgotten by people who trip down the agreeable primrose path to adultery. First, there may well be a good chance that the affair will result in a woman becoming pregnant by the wrong husband. And secondly, there's always the risk that if your fellow-frolicker in bed is promiscuous, you may wind up with a sexual infection – which you may pass on to your spouse.

Having said all that, I have to admit that people are only human and that they do very often stray from the path of virtue – and frequently get away with it. Adultery is incredibly common these days, even in staid, respectable Britain, it seems likely according to recent surveys that:

three out of 10 wives have committed adultery

half of these have had multiple lovers

at any given time, about one in 10 wives is having an affair.

So if you *are* unwise enough to give in to temptation, what's the best way to manage things and keep the situation from getting out of control? Here are some pointers:

firstly, try to bring the affair to an end if you can – the longer it goes on the more the likelihood of trouble

just because you slipped between the sheets with somebody *once* in a moment of weakness doesn't mean you have to do it again

try at all cost not to turn a sexual affair into a genuine love (i.e. loving) affair. There's a tendency for people who fall into bed out of sheer lust to decide before long that they love each other – and that really can be bad news

laughably simple though it sounds, make sure someone is taking contraceptive precautions. You really are going to mess up a marriage (perhaps two marriages) if it looks as though there's going to be a little cuckoo in the nest

if there's the chance that your frolic might have led to infection then for heaven's sake have a confidential check-up at a clinic. It would be totally unfair to give an infection to your innocent spouse – which often happens

finally, unless there's some really overwhelming reason why you have to, *don't confess*. Few people want to be told that their partner has two-timed them: if you *must* confess to someone, see a priest, doctor or marriage guidance counsellor.

Q **How can I get myself out of this difficult situation? I have somehow or other drifted into affairs with two men.**

The big problem is that they are both 'family'. One is my husband's sister's brother-in-law, and the other is my husband's cousin.

A I suppose that's what they call 'sexual relations', is it?

Seriously, adultery is nearly always a dangerous business. Committing adultery with a man who you're related to is *very* dangerous. And doing it with TWO men who you're related to is stark raving bonkers!

I don't want to sound unsympathetic, but I'm always a bit baffled by these letters from people who say 'I'm in an unwise sexual liaison; what do I do?'

The only sane course if you're embroiled in a risky adulterous relationship is to stop it right away! In your case, you need to tell both of these blokes that in future, the only crumpet they'll be getting from you will be on the end of a toasting-fork.

Q **I am 21, have a young child, and have always enjoyed a good sex life with my husband. But recently he accused me of having an affair, because he claims my vagina has expanded and become too big for him. I have always been faithful to him, so this accusation hurts me.**

A I'm sure it does. His idiotic suspicions stem from the common male belief that frequent sexual intercourse enlarges a woman's vagina. This is a ludicrous myth, but you'd be surprised how many men believe it. (There's a well-known 'joke' about a tart who offers to pay a taxi driver by letting him look up her skirt; he eyes her doubtfully, and then says: 'Haven't you got anything smaller?')

Anyway, the only common reason for a vagina being too loose is not lovemaking, but childbirth. I'd suggest you have a check-up from a GP, family planning clinic MO, or gynaecologist, who will tell you whether your vagina needs 'tightening up' with a repair operation, or whether a course of exercise would suffice.

See also **PELVIC FLOOR**

Q **What do you think I should do? I am married, but I have somehow slipped into an affair with a man at our local squash club. It all happened when the two of us played a practice**

game together at the club one afternoon. We seemed to get on awfully well on the court, and we laughed together a lot during the game.

There was no-one else in the building at the time. As the men's and the women's changing rooms are next to each other, we continued chatting to one another through the communicating door.

Just after I'd stepped under the shower, I heard him come up behind me. He took me in his arms, and that was that.

Since then, we have gone on making love at the club during the day when it is quiet. Am I mad to go on with this relationship?

A Squash has always had a bit of a reputation as a sexy sort of game. Maybe that's because of the very close physical contact of fairly scantily-dressed men and women in an enclosed space. As the Americans say, 'Nothing propinks like propinquity.'

Also, there's a theory that when males and females perspire, they give off 'pheromones' – scents which are strong sexual attractants, with a powerful effect on the unconscious mind.

Add to all this the heady brew of an 'unchaperoned' building plus adjacent changing rooms and a warm, soapy shower – and you've got a recipe for disaster.

Honestly, ma'am: if you go on meeting this man in this fashion, it's a hundred to one that somebody is going to find out. The news will get to your husband – and to this bloke's wife (if he has one).

So I urge you to join another squash club – or perhaps change to a different sport altogether.

Furthermore, if anybody catches the pair of you in the club showers, your lover is very likely to end up being blackballed (if you'll forgive the phrase).

Q **My husband wants me to have anal sex during period times when we can't make love in the ordinary way. But what infections can be passed on?**

A Well, AIDS – if, of course, one partner has the HIV virus.

Also, the man can get a urinary infection from the germs in the woman's bowel. And if he were unwise enough to have vaginal intercourse with her immediately afterwards this could give her a vaginal discharge.

Recent work among male gays does suggest that rectal practices, including anal intercourse and kissing ('rimming') do transmit hepatitis, amoebiasis, and an odd form of diarrhoea called 'the gay bowel syndrome'.

Anorgasmia

Anorgasmia means 'inability to reach orgasm', and it is quite common in women, as both my postbag and Dr Kinsey's statistics demonstrate.

Kinsey found that roughly one woman in ten can't reach a climax at all. Many others find considerable difficulty in doing so, and are very worried by this.

But I think that many men and women expect too much of female orgasmic ability.

Many men – especially younger blokes – think that if they have intercourse with a woman, she should automatically and swiftly reach orgasm.

Many younger women think that orgasm should start happening as soon as a girl loses her virginity.

These assumptions are nonsense! Unlike male orgasm, female orgasm isn't almost automatic. It usually needs care, tenderness and skill to produce one – and some women may need an hour or so of stimulation before they are warmed up enough to 'come'.

The ability to reach orgasm is surprisingly low in younger women. According to Kinsey, only about 40% of 20-years-olds can reach an orgasm at all. The ability to have a climax increases rapidly with age, however, and the vast majority of 40-plus women can do it.

So what do you do if you really are having big trouble reaching a climax?

Well, the first thing to clear up is that lack of orgasm is unlikely to have a physical cause and the emotional reasons are many and complex – involving such things as childhood repressions, bad sexual experiences and stress.

One common cause, however, is lack of knowledge. Your man has to know that he is stimulating you in the way that *you* want, and that means you telling him.

Still no luck? Then my advice would be to go to a Family Planning Clinic and ask to see a doctor who has been trained in the 'Balint' or 'Seminar' method of marital therapy. These doctors (mainly women) are adept at helping people unravel the tensions which so often prevent them from reaching orgasm.

An alternative would be to ask your doctor to refer you and your partner to a 'behaviourist' or Masters-Johnson type clinic where the therapists achieve good results in 're-educating', couples who are in difficulties with their sex lives.

Finally, there are a few feminist

groups which attempt to combat anorgasmia through frank mutual 'workshops' and the guided use of self-masturbation and vibrators.

Male anorgasmia

Blokes have this problem too – though nowhere near as commonly as women do. As is the case with most sexual problems, physical causes are uncommon.

However, certain widely-prescribed medications (particularly for high blood pressure) can cause difficulty in reaching orgasm. So too can alcohol.

Men who have had prostate surgery may also experience problems reaching a climax – though here the difficulty is often the fact that the man's ejaculate (that is, his fluid) is 'shot' backwards into his urinary bladder rather than outwards. Unfortunately, nothing much can be done about this – though if the couple want to have children, it is technically possible to collect the sperms from his urine, and then inseminate them into his wife.

A common cause of failure to reach orgasm is simply *tiredness* – often combined with stress. Regrettably, a lot of chaps these days are too proud to admit thay they're a bit too tired (or too uptight) to reach a climax. As a result, we're now seeing the extraordinary new phenomenon of *men* faking orgasm.

Obviously, the remedy in these cases is to try to get to bed earlier. If you're still too tired then, at the end of the day set the alarm for an earlier time than you need in the morning. Alternatively make love out of bed and away from the bedroom which is strongly associated with sleep. Also, be frank with your partner, talk things over with her – and try and relax and take life easier. If these commonsense measures fail, then it's wise to seek professional counselling.

There's a large group of men who suffer from what the Americans have grandly termed 'ejaculatory incompetence'.

They have perfectly normal male hormones, but something (most probably inhibitions from early in life) makes it very difficult for them to actually go over the top and reach orgasm.

They usually enjoy love-making, and are often popular with female partners – for the obvious reason that they tend to go on for hours and hours. While this can be pleasurable for the women in their lives, there usually comes a time when a couple decide that 'something's got to be done about it'!

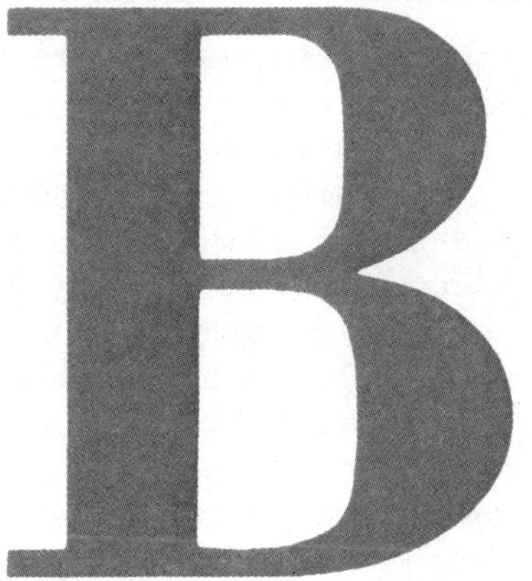

Bereavement

Unfortunately, one person in virtually every loving couple has eventually to face bereavement from their partner – sometimes tragically early.

If this happens to *you* early in life, it's absolutely devastating. Many people feel like killing themselves – and a few do.

But the fact is that most people who are bereaved early in their married lives do (often much to their amazement) manage to get things back on an even keel. Many of them do eventually start going out with other people – and a lot get married again. Such marriages are often highly successful – though you should *never* rush into one just 'to give the children a father/mother'. As you're doubtless well aware, almost all stepchildren are wary of (and potentially hostile toward) any stepfather or stepmother.

A far more common situation, of course, is for a loving couple to survive 30 or 40 years together, and then to be split up by death quite *late* in life. Though it's common, it doesn't make it easier to bear.

I get a lot of letters from people who've recently been bereaved. The main hope I can offer is something every doctor knows: that eventually most of them *do* find a purpose in living, particularly through their interest in their children and grandchildren. Some who have *no* children find fulfilment in helping others.

What about the sexual aspect of bereavement? I receive an amazing number of letters from people who have lost their partners – but who still have very strong sexual feelings. Most of these letters are from women – which is partly a reflection of the fact that women tend to outlive men.

Obviously, it can be very distressing if you're a widow of 65 or 70 and you find that you're still troubled by strong sexual urges (a common situation judging by my postbag). I think the first thing to say is that – in answer to a question frequently raised by grannies (!) who write to my column – yes it's perfectly acceptable to relieve these tensions by masturbation.

However the fact is (however awful it may sound to someone who's recently been bereaved), *you're never too old to get married again*. Many people who've had happy and loving marriages, and who eventually lose their loved ones, do later remarry at 65 or 70. I've even seen people remarry at 90 – which gives one fresh hope, I must say!

Finally, I would like to stress that there is an encouraging new trend in the development of organizations which counsel those who've lost their loved ones. There are bodies like the Compassionate Friends in Britain, or Cruse, who try to help people through the cruel loss of the person they have loved for life.

Q I am under great stress, as I have discovered after 25 years of marriage that my husband has felt the need to find new friends from 'the gay community'. I try to keep the house nice and myself attractive, but I know that he can barely touch me – although I realise that he must have some spark of love left, because he is still very generous with his gifts. Could he be bisexual?

A I'm afraid this is very possible. Indeed, the poor man may have discovered that he's really homosexual, rather than

Bisexuality

Although many people find the whole idea incomprehensible and distasteful, it's undeniable that a good many 'happily married' husbands and wives are bisexual – in other words, they have the urge to obtain sexual pleasure from both men and women.

My eyes were opened to this fact years ago when I worked in a busy VD clinic – where we'd see Mr Jones, respectable banker and father of four, who just *happened* to have a boyfriend in Chelsea. Since then, the bisexual lives of rather a lot of famous people have been revealed, and we've actually reached the extraordinary stage where some pop stars seemed to revel in it.

However, finding that your partner is bisexual is no fun (as Mrs Oscar Wilde discovered). Quite apart from anything else, if the bisexual partner is male there is the everpresent danger of bringing infections – possibly even AIDS – into the home.

Astonishingly though, I have encountered some cases in which a loving spouse was somehow or other willing to make an effort to cope with his or her partner's bisexuality, and make a go of the marriage. This was, of course, the case with the celebrated and eccentric partnership of Harold Nicolson and Vita Sackville-West.

bisexual. I say 'the poor man' because I'm sure he's as distressed as you are by the crisis that has hit your marriage. In fact, this is an increasingly common situation these days: you'd be surprised at the number of husbands who suddenly realise that they're gay. I think that the pair of you have got to come to a decision as to whether you want the marriage to go on. I have known women who made a success of a marriage with a gay or bisexual husband, but it certainly isn't easy. I'm afraid you have to face the fact that a divorce might eventually turn out to be the best solution – especially if, as you say, your husband no longer wants physical contact with you. However, all is not yet lost – there is a 'Relate' Marriage Guidance Clinic in the city from which you write, and I think you should see them – *rapidly*. It'd also be worth getting in touch with the Albany Trust Counselling, *24 Chester Square, London SW1 9JF*, who have great experience in dealing with the social and emotional problems faced by homosexuals – and indeed by the wives of homosexuals.

Q Your frankness and sense of humour in SHE are refreshing, but I really do not understand why you condemn 'kinky' sex games involving bondage.

I am a divorcée with two sons, and we live with my slightly younger boyfriend. My man will sometimes tie me to the bed before making love to me. Or sometimes he will put me across his knee and spank me. I am quite a dominant woman normally, so being 'dominated' in this way can be quite exciting!

A Whatever turns you on, ma'am. All I'm saying is that bondage games do occasionally lead to nasty accidents – which have, on rare occasions, proved fatal. But it doesn't sound as though you two are into anything involving gags, or ropes round the neck.

I also think that women should run a mile if they meet a guy who wants to introduce real sadism into the bedroom. But I do agree with you that your bit of bottom-smacking isn't hurting anyone or anything (except possibly your *derrière*).

The female bottom

The female bottom has always been a subject of great interest to the male sex – as any woman who has ever endured the indignity of a stroll along the Via Veneto will know. But the buttocks are undoubtedly an erogenous zone of the body – so much so that some women can reach orgasm through having their bottoms patted or even slapped. The are so many sexually-tuned nerve endings in that area of the body that a firm stimulus – like gentle slapping – is bound to fire off a few sensual circuits in the nervous system.

It also has to be admitted that the anal area is even more rich with sexually-tuned nerve endings. This is why anal love-play ('postillionage') and even anal intercourse are so common. A *Playboy* sex survey indicated that a rather alarming 54% of those couples who took part in the survey had tried anal sex. I say 'alarming' because of the hygiene risks of this practice.

The male bottom

As with the female bottom, the male one is a sexually arousable area. In other words, most men like having their buttocks caressed. And as with some women, some men also like having it gently slapped or spanked. With a minority of men, this seems to go a great deal further: in other words, they actually enjoy being caned, even though it hurts a good deal. I cannot account for this male tendency but it seems to be a very widespread one. There may be something in the well known theory that all these men have been deeply influenced by the repeated bottom canings they experienced at school. (But since corporal punishment has become so rare in recent years, it's surprising that the trend has not died out.) There is certainly no harm in a little honest bottom smacking in bed, but there is no point in going in for it unless you really want to.

The other extremely sexual area of the male bottom is the anus. Just as is the case with the female back passage this is a region where there appear to be a lot of erotic nerve endings. A lot of people think that it's only homosexual males who get sexual pleasure in this way but that is not true. In Britain, the USA and many other western countries, it has become the smart thing for sophisticated women to slip a lubricated finger inside the man's rectum while making love, or having oral sex. However, there seem to me to be real risks in doing it, if you're not *very* careful about washing your hands immediately afterwards. In particular, some of the alarming 'new' sexual infections which are spreading across the world may well be transmitted by this sort of play.

Finally, let me add that there is one other quite common way of stimulating the male (or indeed female) bottom. This is with the 'rectal vibrators' which are widely sold in sex shops. I mention these only to say that *you should not use them*. Vaginal vibrators are quite a different thing, but rectal vibrators can sometimes vanish inside you!

Q I have very small breasts. My girl friend wants me to go to a 'non-textile' (ie nudist) beach with her this summer. Do you think I will feel embarrassed?

A Probably. I speak from personal experience – because some time back, I reported on a naturist camp for a medical magazine, and had to strip off to conduct the interviews. However, I can tell you that the embarrassment tends to last about two minutes flat – by which time you've realised that no-one is paying any attention to the size and shape of your personal bits and pieces.

By the bye, I found that naturists were a jolly and friendly lot. They run things like sponsored nude swims in aid of leukaemia. And the organiser of their Singles Club keeps writing to me to say that they need lots more female members. Interested readers should write to CCBN, Assurance House, *35–41 Hazelwood Rd, Northampton NN1 1LL* for a leaflet called Bare With Us!

See also **THE NIPPLE**

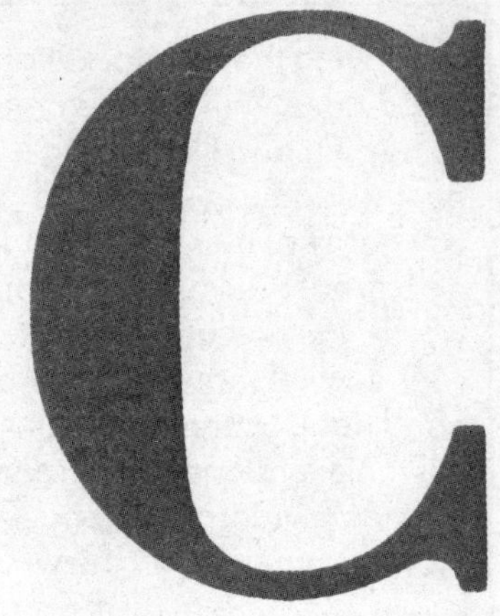

Q I am that modern-day rarity, a 23-year-old-virgin. I believe I am an attractive, intelligent and confident woman with no hang-ups about my sexuality. I'm a virgin for religious and moral reasons.

I have a very loving boyfriend, and everything in my life would be perfect, if it were not for my past.

From the age of 14 to 20, I was cajoled by my father into performing various sexual acts with him (I always refused full intercourse). I complied out of love for him, and because I was able to sense his desperation.

He died two years ago, and now I have real emotional happiness with my boyfriend.

My dilemma lies in whether or not I should tell him about my father?

A First of all, I must congratulate you on your immensely courageous letter.

From the unpublished part of it, I gather that you've never told a living soul about your Dad, and feel it would be 'betraying his secret' to talk directly to someone about what he did.

Mainly for that reason, I don't think you should tell your boyfriend – *yet*. It would be better to kick off by speaking to an anonymous individual, who is experienced in dealing with the problems caused by incest.

So please ring the *Incest Crisis* line – on either *01–422 5100* or *01–890 4732*. Their counsellors will, I'm sure, help you lift the burden of the past from your shoulders. Good luck.

Q After 16 years of marriage, my wife has just horrified me by telling me that she wants to rub her own clitoris during intercourse. This has really shaken me.

Should she really *need* this sort of thing?

A Well, I'm sorry if your poor old ego was a bit wounded by your missus' revelation!

But there's no need for alarm. You see, vast numbers of women *do* need clitoral stimulation during sexual intercourse. And my analysis of the returns from a *Delvin Report* shows that many **SHE** readers do actually *give themselves* that stimulation – at the same time as their menfolk make love to them.

Unfortunately, a lot of men just can't handle this (so to speak). But I think you should just regard it as a natural part of your wife's sexuality – and be glad she's happy.

See also **MASTURBATION**

Clitoral Stimulation

In just the same way as the penis, the clitoris becomes erect during sexual excitement – either as a result of thinking erotic thoughts, or as a result of direct stimulation.

And as is the case with the penis, the clitoris becomes erect simply because it fills up with blood – so that it becomes stiffer.

People do get rather the wrong idea about erection of the clitoris. They've usually read about it in sex manuals or school biology books, and think that the clitoris is going to turn into something like a small courgette!

But in fact your clitoris is a very tiny organ indeed. It's only about the size of a baked bean, and most of it is internal so that from the outside, you can only see a little 'bump' about the size of a shirt button.

Even during sexual excitement, the external part is only about half the size of a processed pea, so that it just peeks out from under the 'hood'.

However, this amount of erection does seem to bring it more firmly into contact with the man's pubic region – which is very important if the woman is to achieve satisfaction.

Q **I'm pregnant and find my sexual feelings much stronger than before – I have to rub my clitoris at night. Will this harm the baby?**

A Not at all, ma'am particularly as your clitoris is away from where the baby is. If this innocent practice helps you relax and to cope better with your pregnancy – just lie back and enjoy it.

Q **Could my umbilicus be connected to my clitoris? My friends think I'm mad, but I wonder if my belly button is an erogenous zone? Certainly, when my fiancé rubs it, I can virtually reach a climax.**

A I've heard of naval manoeuvres, but this is ridiculous! If your letter isn't a hoax, then my conclusion is simply that you are remarkably lucky. (And so is your fiancé . . .)

Clitoris

One of the unexpected bonuses of being lucky enough to have your books translated into foreign languages is that you find out all sorts of useful foreign words.

In German, it's *die Kitzler,* in Dutch its *de clitoris,* in French it's *le cli-cli* and in Hebrew its represented by something that looks like the figures '72727' followed by a picture of Stonehenge.

So there's a lot of interest in the clitoris all over the world. Regrettably, in Britain lots of men and women aren't too clear about just where the clitoris is or what it does. This is a pity, because it is the main key to sexual pleasure in most women.

Because so many couples are vague about the location and function of the clitoris, their sex lives are often frustrating and unhappy. Once they *do* find out where it is – and what to do with it – things often improve dramatically.

A woman's clitoris is located just in front of her pubic bone – so that with a bit of luck, it will be gently compressed and squeezed between the man's pubes and her own during intercourse.

It's only about the same width as a little blouse button – even when it swells up during sexual excitement. But close examination reveals that it is almost identical in structure to a man's penis. So it's not surprising that it's more plentifully supplied with pleasure-producing nerve-endings than any other part of the female body.

I haven't space to embark on description of the many possible clitoris-stimulation techniques. But male readers may like to note the point that during love-play, many lasses (not all) do prefer to be stimulated along the *side* of the clitoris, rather than directly on top of it.

Disorders of the clitoris are rare. Occasionally women seek medical advice because of a sudden and alarming swelling of the clitoris. This swelling appears to be due to a collection of blood – and it soon bursts, leaving no ill-effects.

Some years ago, I described the condition in the doctors' magazine *World Medicine,* and promptly received a number of letters from practitioners who had seen it. Two of them mentioned cases in which the woman had actually caused the swelling by wrapping a cotton thread round her clitoris during masturbation – clearly, this is *not* a sensible idea.

Q Help, help, help! My fiancé and I have been using the condom as our means of contraception, but we've had three of the said objects burst on us! I thought that these wonderful 'AIDS-preventing' condoms had stringent tests?

A They do, they do – not only electronic tests but also being filled with water and being dropped from a great height!

However, the fact is that the public (both male and female) like condoms to be sensitive – and that means very thin indeed. So inevitably, there will be times when even a completely flawless condom will tear.

You can minimise the chances of this happening by:

(a) following the instructions on the manufacturer's leaflet to the letter (or even the French letter).
(b) Taking great care to avoid nicking the sheath with fingernails, engagement rings – or even teeth.

But if the condoms continue to burst, it could be due to the fact that your fiancé is . . . er . . . a very big lad. In which case you may possibly wish to switch to another method. (British manufacturers do not make specially big condoms – they're all one size).

One final point for all condom-users out there. The Family Planning Association does recommend that women protect themselves against the risk of a burst condom by using a vaginal spermicidal pessary as well. You can buy these without embarrassment at chemist's – and in Family Planning Clinics, where they're usually given out in the same pack as the condoms.

Condom Allergy

There's good news for those couples who can't use sheaths because of an allergy. Durex have launched a new, lubricated hypo-allergenic sheath, simply (if unimaginatively) called 'Durex Allergy'.

I must say that if I were a bloke who had an allergy to French letters, I'd certainly prefer these new condoms to the alternative answer, which is to use a sheath made not of rubber, but of lambs' intestines (yuk).

Q I'm due to be married next Easter, and my fiancé has just told me he likes dressing up in women's clothes. What do I do?

A I'm sure this has come as a big shock to you. But there are many 'cross-dressers' around. Rather surprisingly, quite a lot of them do make happy and successful marriages – though their wives have to be pretty understanding.

One possible factor in the success of some of these marriages is that quite a few women do seem to get a kick out of seeing men dressed up in women's clothing, though I don't know why.

But I think you must go very carefully during the next few months. Talk this over very thoroughly with your fiancé before you agree to go ahead with the wedding. You *must* ask him whether he has homosexual or bisexual leanings – though in fact, many transvestites are basically heterosexual.

Even if you love the guy very much, I think you might do better to live with him for a while, before you actually tie the nuptial knot with someone who may be borrowing your knickers for the next 60 years. Good luck.

Cross Dressing

Most people assume that because transvestites like dressing up in 'drag', they must be homosexual. But the spokesperson for their organisation says that nearly all the gents who belong to his society are very much heterosexual – and often married too.

I'm inclined to believe him. Some years ago, the medical journal for which I work despatched a woman reporter to cover a conference for transvestite men.

Afterwards, she indignantly reported that one of them had tried to grope her in the back of a taxi – despite the fact that he was wearing diamanté earrings and evening gown!

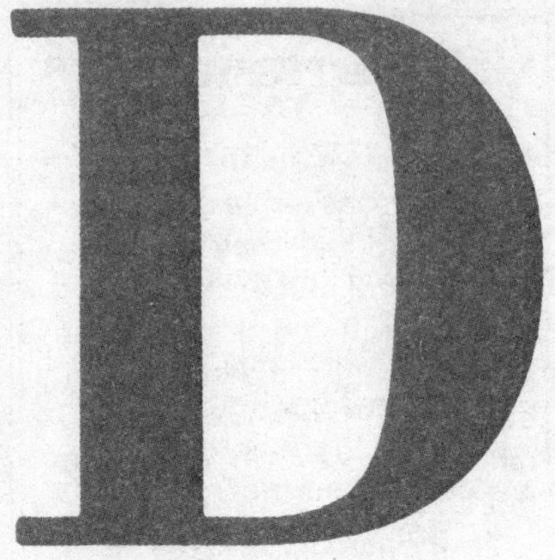

Q I am a divorcée, heading for 40, lonely but still quite attractive. Last summer I went on a sailing holiday in Greece and much to my surprise had a tremendously satisfying affair with a young Greek courier.

Now he has written to me, inviting me to come sailing with him this summer in the Aegean. Do you think I'd be crazy to renew this relationship with a man who is about half my age?

A I don't think you'd be crazy at all, ma'am. Sailing in Greece provides a tremendous holiday (even if – like Cap'n Delvin last year – you very nearly scuppered your yacht in the wine-dark sea!).

If you, as a lonely, 40-ish divorcée, can combine a sailing holiday in that beautiful country with a satisfying emotional and physical relationship provided by some young Apollo, then good luck to you.

One shouldn't always beware the Greeks when they come bearing (or indeed, baring) gifts . . .

Divorce

It's a pretty awful thought that (in most western societies) at least one in three of all those who get married will some day have to face marriage breakdown.

It's tragic, but those are the facts. I get more and more depressed when I read the divorce statistics each year!

Although there are variations between countries, it seems that almost everywhere, the trend towards divorce is on the increase. Repeated divorce – or 'serial monogamy', as they call it in California, has now become quite socially acceptable.

Britain is fairly typical of most western societies: 80% of all divorces occur in first marriages. Which means, if you think about it, that one in five of all divorces involves somebody for whom this was already the second marriage!

Indeed, in nearly one in 10 cases, *both husband and wife* have been married before, and are going through their second divorce. This lends new weight to Dr Johnson's famous statement that second marriages represent 'a triumph of hope over experience'!

Obviously, I can only hope to deal in this book with the sexual side of coping with a divorce. But if divorce does strike your marriage, how are *you* going to cope with it sexually?

The first thing to say is this. *Don't assume that your love-life is over!*

Although I've said that a second marriage should be regarded with caution, there's no reason to feel that matrimony is 'out' for you from now on.

Nor are enjoyable romantic relationships with the opposite sex by any means over. It's very easy for a divorced person – particularly a woman – to think, ''My love-life is finished.' But that's not necessarily true: life still holds plenty of romance – and *divorcées* (and *divorcés* too) are socially very much in demand these days!

Indeed, the problem for both *divorcée* and *divorcé* may be quite the reverse. Enthusiastic would-be lovers tend to swarm round any recently divorced person who is even half-way attractive, and there may be very real difficulty in keeping all these characters out of your bed!

I have to say that there's a terrible tendency among many newly-divorced people (both men and women) to give in to the temptation to partake 'not wisely, but too well' of all these offers. I have received in my postbag a fairly typical letter from a recently-divorced woman who had been quite 'bowled over' to find out, after all these years of monogamy, that she was highly attractive to men.

The poor lady had (according to her letter) slept with all the handsome men who flocked round her, and had (I quote) 'a fantastic time', as she discovered that most of them were far better lovers than her husband. This experience is common.

Unfortunately, in the end (literally) she got herpes. Naturally, she was now pretty distraught. She'd been particularly distressed at the idea that she'd 'never be able to make love again' – which fortunately isn't really true.

This kind of wild over-indulgence often occurs after divorce. It may result in:

sexual infection

emotional hurt

unwanted pregnancy

difficulties with existing children – who may understandably be very upset that a parent keeps coming home with a replacement Daddy or Mummy on Saturday nights.

So, play it a bit cool. *Don't* rush headlong into unwise affairs. *Do* remember that contraception is (usually) still necessary. *Do* remember that one-night stands tend to bring infection. And above all, bear in mind that *you must not let your love-life upset your children*.

However, never forget that you do still have a chance of finding a life-long loving relationship. Despite Sam Johnson's dictum about repeat marriages, they do very often succeed. Why, you've only to look at Ronald Reagan and Nancy!

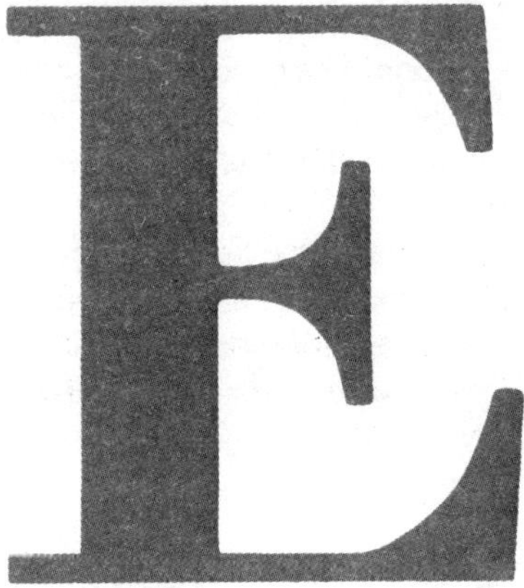

Q I have been told that for a man to 'hold back' when he feels ejaculation coming on is dangerous and may cause internal injury, is this true?

A No, I think this is a myth. There was a time when certain naturopaths used to suggest that 'holding back' could cause enlargement of the prostate in later life. But there's no medical evidence whatever for this.

In practice, it would be very difficult for a man to be any kind of a decent lover unless he learned to postpone his climax, in order to prolong his partner's enjoyment.

Q My boyfriend has asked me to write to you about the subject of female ejaculation, because he says you know about it.

I thought I was abnormal when I first did it at a climax, and felt terribly ashamed. But he says it is normal. Is this true? And if so, what is the fluid which I produce at the moment of orgasm?

A Your boyfriend is quite right. Surprisingly, it's normal for some women to squirt out a fluid at the moment of orgasm. This usually causes them great distress until they eventually find out that it's OK.

Along with most other docs, I used to believe that this fluid was always urine – and that the ladies were being slightly incontinent under the wholly understandable stress of 'coming'!

But research in America has suggested very strongly that it's actually a special sex fluid, rather similar to the secretion which is ejaculated from a man's prostate gland, but produced by a sensitive structure near the famous G-spot. (That G-spot gets everywhere these days, doesn't it?)

Actually, I'm not yet totally convinced by the US research on the chemical nature of this liquid, but (as far as I know) no-one this side of the Atlantic has tried to analyse it.

A **SHE** reader did once attempt to send me a sample of her fluid, but most unfortunately the bottle broke in the post with disastrous results!

See also **THE G-SPOT; ORGASM; THE VAGINA**

Q You seem to get quite a lot of letters about premature ejaculation. Well, my husband's trouble is the opposite.

In fact, he simply cannot 'come'. He can have sex with me, but during the five years we've been together, he has only ejaculated twice.

On those two occasions he only managed it after a marathon effort of interminable 'bonking', which was very sore and painful for me.

A Sorry to hear about this. Your husband's problem is called 'ejaculatory incompetence', and there's quite a bit of it about. Cause is unknown, but thought to be emotional.

Happily, the old behaviourist firm of Masters and Johnson have a system of 're-training' which usually does the trick. It would involve you – and you'd need to be prepared to spend many hours in the type of activity usually undertaken by topless masseuses.

Not all wives are willing to do this but your letter gives me the impression that you are keen to help your man overcome (sorry) his disability.

Now you need a therapist to teach you both the re-training programme. Please give the Family Planning Service a ring on 01-636-7866, and they'll be able to give you the nearest one.

See also **ANORGASMIA**

Engagement

Being engaged can be either a very happy or a very difficult time. Unfortunately, there are often stresses from all sides – from parents, relatives, friends and (if it's a second marriage – as it often is these days) from former wives and/or husbands!

There are also difficult financial pressures – unless you're very rich! There can be tricky social obligations, with the need to keep all sorts of people happy.

And there's the major stress (at least, it's a major stress for a lot of people) of having to be the central actors in that emotion-charged theatrical event: a wedding. No wonder so many brides (and grooms) do a bunk.

The important things to remember during an engagement:

1. Be patient with your partner – because he or she is probably under a lot of stress too.
2. Be nice to your partner's family (even if it's the ex-wife or ex-husband!). The family bitterness that so frequently arises at or before a wedding will all too often last a lifetime.
3. If you become doubtful about marriage, *for heaven's sake put it off*! It doesn't matter what arrangements have been made or how much money will be lost (it doesn't even matter if you're pregnant): the fact is that you should never embark on the frail ship of matrimony unless you're absolutely *sure* that this is the sailor you want to spend the rest of the voyage with. Because the rest of the voyage is *life*.
4. Similarly, if the two of you seem to be sexually incompatible – or if one or other of you has serious sex problems – then think very carefully before going ahead with the wedding. Far too many people think that 'it'll be all right when we're married.' It probably won't.

Q Sex with my husband is super, but – embarrassingly for him – he does tend to lose his erection a little, about half way through intercourse. Is there anything we can do about this?

A A common problem, ma'am. In fact, there's a simple solution, providing the difficulty is relatively mild.

Next time you're making love with him, slip your hand down

Erection

The function of erection is rather vital to the survival of the human race.

First of all, can I make the point that it's important for women to realise that most men tend to be a bit obsessed with this particular human function. Which is not surprising, really – because it's very difficult and frustrating and embarrassing for a bloke if erection doesn't happen when wanted.

The actual stiffening of the penis is caused by a dramatic increase in blood flow into the three hollow chambers which make up most of the organ.

But what makes the male organ become engorged with blood like this? It's a complicated interaction between three different areas of the human nervous system, one of which has been discovered by Professor Julia Polak and her colleagues at Hammersmith Hospital.

This new area of the nervous system works by releasing a chemical with the unlikely name of VIP (it stands for vasoactive intestinal polypeptide.)

Research in Britain, Denmark and France shows that some impotent men are lacking in VIP and if you inject it into a man's penis, he will develop an erection. So there are some hopes that it'll eventually be possible to manufacture the stuff as a cure for impotence.

However, under ordinary circumstances, there are two different factors which will give a man an erection. They are (a) thinking about sex (b)direct rubbing or stroking of his penis.

It seems that in some way, these activities release the above-mentioned VIP into the man's phallus, and to help make it erect.

Now it's absolutely vital for any woman to realise that activity (a) above – ie 'thinking about sex' – may well not be enough to give a male an erection, particularly if he's nervous or tired, or perhaps not quite as young as he was.

Yes – contrary to what you might think from reading certain popular novels, quite a few men don't 'leap to attention' as soon as their beloved starts taking her clothes off!

So the point I'm making is that many chaps do need quite a lot of activity (b), mentioned above, before they're in a fit state to make love.

So there it is, dear readers: very often the future of your man's potency is quite literally in your hands . . .

between your two tums (so to speak) and hold him, firmly but agreeably, stimulating with your fingers as necessary.

If more wives knew this simple ploy, far fewer gents would have probs with potency.

Q I'm 67, and my husband is 70, and he's having trouble satisfying me these days. This is because his erection is so unreliable.

Are there any drugs (private or NHS) which would enable him to become erect, even if it was only once or twice a month?

A Yes, there are now. But I must stress that your husband ought to talk this problem over carefully with your doc – and have a physical examination – before any decision is made as to whether to use these VERY powerful drugs. They have to be injected directly into the penis just before sex, and they can have rather drastic side-effects (like, for instance, an erection that simply won't go down unless a surgeon removes blood from the engorged organ).

For that reason, the injection treatment is as a rule prescribed by urological surgeons, rather than by GPs.

Exercise and Sex

Recently there have been persistent suggestions in the newspapers that exercise is somehow bad for you sexually. But what are the facts?

Well, earlier this year I was fortunate enough to chair a sports medicine symposium at which one of the speakers was medical officer to the British women's team in a certain sport. (For obvious reasons, I won't say *which* sport . . .)

He revealed that the intensive training which these international sportswomen go in for has one little-known side-effect. Virtually none of them have periods.

It appears that heavy and repeated exercise (for instance, running 50 or so miles a week is likely to stop a woman's periods. Some top sports-women haven't had 'the curse' for years.

Fortunately, the effect seems to be only *temporary*, and it's thought that most sportswomen get their periods back when they stop training.

And what about their love-lives? As far as I can discover, although many top sportswomen don't menstruate they still have a perfectly healthy interest in sex. A high proportion feel it wisest to take the pill (since the absence of periods *doesn't* mean that you can't get pregnant).

Indeed, it's rumoured that in a recent British women's sports team, every member but one was on the pill. The odd one out turned out to be a man.

What about the effect of exercise on *blokes'* sex lives?

I've noticed a lot of reports in the media which claim that jogging causes impotence. Indeed, when I was doing a radio phone-in recently I was *assured* by the presenter that this anti-erotic effect of jogging had been proved by an American university. 'They've shown that it lowers your male hormone levels' he told me.

Well I've got good news for anxious joggers. In fact, the whole thing was an April Fools' Day hoax in my own medical newspaper *General Practitioner*!

Unfortunately, the hoax was swallowed hook, line and sinker by a national paper, and it's been constantly repeated since then.

But I can assure you, gents – the only way that jogging will make you limp is if you twist your ankle!

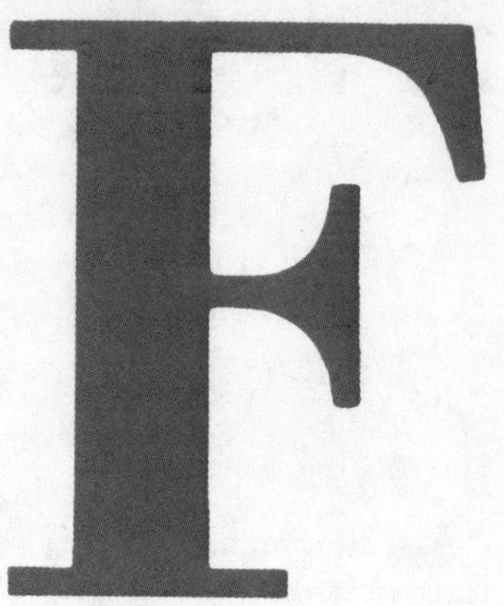

Q **For how long are men supposed to provide women with foreplay?**

I ask because I really am getting rather tired of providing this service for my wife. Sometimes she wants as much as 15 minutes before I'm allowed to have intercourse with her.

A Well sir, I've recently come across an American sex survey in which a large number of US ladies were asked: 'How long do you usually like loveplay to last?'

The answers (which may shatter you somewhat) were as follows:

less than five minutes	2 per cent
five to fifteen minutes	36 per cent
up to half an hour	48 percent
up to an hour	14 per cent

So, many women prefer up to 30 minutes of love play – and some want up to an hour. Your poor old missus is being relatively undemanding in only asking for up to 15 minutes.

Frankly, the general tone of your question is so selfish that it makes me a bit dubious about the prospects for your marriage. I suggest you rapidly review your attitude to your wife's sexual and emotional needs – before she starts looking for love play elsewhere.

See also LOVE PLAY

Q **I read what you said about the survey that showed so many women wanted lots of foreplay.**

Now I really think I'm odd, because I don't like it at all. I'm 38, and happily married with a great sex life. But I like to get right on with it! I hate being petted first. Am I the only one!

A Not at all, ma'am. It looks as though about a few per cent of women are satisfied with less than five minutes of loveplay before intercourse. And a substantial number of them simply can't stand foreplay at all, and just want to get right on with it – like you.

Indeed, marital arts specialists find that when these women come into the consulting room complaining about their sex lives, the best thing to do is to tell their husbands to abandon all attempts at preliminary petting and just charge right in!

Q **I just don't know what to do about my marriage. Several years ago, my wife and I drifted into a foursome with a very nice couple who share our interests in chamber music, opera,**

bridge, ski-ing – and of course sex.

No one else knew that the four of us had this sexual arrangement, and it all seemed very discreet and civilised. But things began to go wrong when we all went ski-ing in Kitzbühl last winter. To be frank, the two wives seemed to get more and more interested in each other, and less and less interested in us.

By the time we came home, they appeared to be very emotionally wrapped up in one another. And now both of them seem to have lost all interest in their marriages, and they are talking about setting up home together.

Have you any suggestions as to what we two husbands should do?

A I'm sorry to hear about this predicament, but I'm not surprised.

In Britain there's been a very strong trend toward these 'discreet' and 'civilised' mixed foursomes ever since the 1960s. Some couples have got away with such arrangements, but many others have hit serious troubles.

What usually happens is that the wife in marriage A falls in love with the husband in marriage B and they go off together, with resultant chaos all round.

Various permutations are possible, but I must admit that your particular situation (with the two wives falling in love with each other during the warm glow of the *après ski*) is a trifle unusual.

So what are you to gents to do? If both your wives are basically lesbian, then I think you've had it.

But I reckon that there's a chance you might be able to win them back if you're willing to try really hard.

This means devoting yourself to trying to romance your wife, and to wooing her back to you single-mindedly. Make clear to her that you love her, and that you'd give anything to have her back again.

Most important of all, tell her that from now on, you want her one-to-one, and not with some other bloke sharing the goodies. Then for heaven's sake, bid this other couple farewell – and don't get involved in any more sexual shenanigans with them.

Q I'm not a nymphomaniac but I do need sex very badly. If I don't get it, I become very edgy.

But I split up from my boyfriend some time back. So what do I do? I refuse to 'sleep around' just to relieve my frustration until Mr Right happens to come along!

A I entirely agree with you. For a highly sexed woman such as yourself, it is much more sensible and safe to rely on masturbation until the right relationship eventually turns up.

Don't feel bad about doing this! One **SHE** survey suggested that a staggering 85 per cent of readers sometimes go in for a spot of 'DIY'. So you'd be in good company, so to speak.

Q I have a good relationship with my husband. However, just after my period finishes each month, I feel very sexually aroused, and want to make love to my husband. Unfortunately, he doesn't share this feeling. He says I'm putting him under pressure, so that he feels like a 'performing animal'. So he just won't reciprocate. This makes me upset and angry, which makes him retreat even more. What can I do?

A Difficult. If this only happens just at the end of your period, I'd say that he's probably one of the many men who aren't totally happy with the fact that women actually menstruate. (The ancient male taboos against having sex with 'menstruous women' are very strong – see the Book of Leviticus). But I think it's more likely that he can't cope with being 'hunted' rather than the 'hunter'.

Either way, I reckon that you both need to sort this out quickly – or your marriage could be heading into trouble. Ask him if he'll go along with you for a chat at 'Relate'; you'll find them in the phone book probably still under their old name – the Marriage Guidance Council.

Q My husband is away in the Merchant Navy for months at a time, and to be frank I get very frustrated sexually.

Recently I have discovered to my surprise that I can ease this frustration by gently playing my hair dryer over my 'pubes'.

Have you any medical objection to this?

A None at all. Better a blow-dry than a boyfriend.

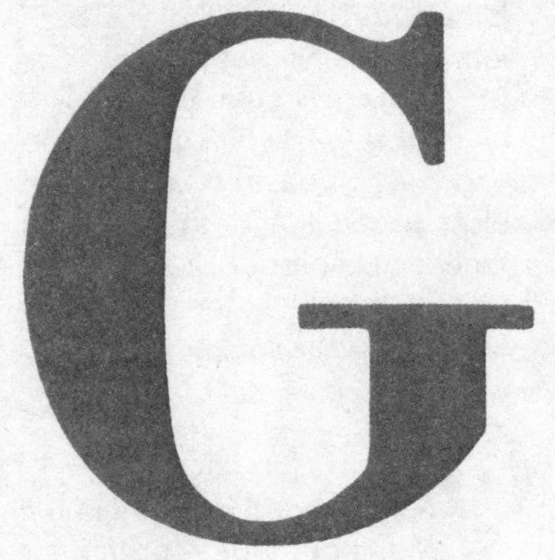

The G-spot

Controversy still rages about whether the 'magic female G-spot' really exists or not. I am inclined to think that it *does* – and that stimulation of it can help some women who have difficulty in getting sexually aroused, or in reaching a climax. It may also be connected with the curious phenomen of 'female ejaculation'.

My knowledge of the G-spot goes back to a time several years ago when I wrote in my column that it was a 'complete myth' that women ejaculated a fluid at the moment of orgasm. I was immediately flooded with protest letters from readers who said that they *did* do this. One lady even sent

Q Where on earth is my blooming G-spot?

My husband and I have tried repeatedly to find it, but no luck at all. We gather it's half-way up the front wall of the vagina, but we just seem to get a bit lost.

Could you print a map?

A Well ma'am, I'm still a bit doubtful whether the Famous Female G-spot really exists – but me a sample of the liquid, but the container broke in the post.

At this stage, two readers wrote to me to point out that an obscure US sexological journal had just published a series of research papers which indicated that women had something called a G-spot (named after its discoverer, Ernst Grafenberg), and that stimulation of this newly-discovered organ could produce a climax – a climax which was sometimes accompanied by a squirt of some mysterious sexual fluid.

It's located in very much the same situation as the male prostate gland, and it's interesting that US and Canadian researchers have claimed that the liquid which it's supposed to produce is in fact very similar in chemical composition to the secretion of the prostate. So it's claimed that the 'G-spot' is a sort of 'homologue' (i.e. an exact anatomical equivalent) of a man's prostate gland.

Not altogether surprisingly, the new 'anti-sex movement' in the USA has been claiming that the G-spot doesn't exist at all. But whether it does or not, searching for it may actually help some women with sexual difficulties. If you or partner gently rub an area about half-way up the front wall of your vagina with a soft fingertip, you'll rapidly be able to draw your own conclusions as to whether the G-spot is real – or just a fig-leaf of somebody's imagination...

I'm inclined to think that there's *something* there, if you can only put your finger on it....

It is claimed that the G-spot is a specially sensitive female organ – the exact equivalent of the male prostate gland.

American sexperts claim that stimulation of it helps women who have difficulty reaching orgasm – and that the climaxes produced by rubbing this spot are more intense than ordinary ones – and may be accompanied by release of some special love-fluid.

My own feeling is that the G-spot may not be a real organ at all – but just a very sensitive area over the urethra (water-pipe) – which is just in front of the vagina.

But how the heck do you find it? Best thing is to wait until love-play has you well-lubricated. Then lie on your tummy on the bed, with your legs well apart.

Your husband should sit beside you, and should gently slip his index and middle fingers into your vagina (palm downwards).

He'll find that he can sort of

'hook' the pads of his fingertips over the shelf-like projection of your pubic bone. Just beyond this is the area of your G-spot. It's undeniable that if he caresses this zone with his fingers, you will experience all sorts of agreeable and unusual sensations.

Well, that's the G-plan! I hope you're all joining in at home . . .

Q Am I abnormal? You see, I read what you said about the 'magic G spot'. I appear to have *five* of these in my vaginal area, all very sexually excitable.

A Lucky old you. No, you're not abnormal. Lots of people have more than one specially sensitive area inside their vagina.

Group Sex

Group sex is very popular these days: you'd be amazed how many discreet orgies are arranged in well-appointed London town houses, or in 'respectable' Californian ranch houses. But everything I've said about the dangers of wife-swapping and open marriages applies with about 50 times more force to group sex.

For a start, the multiplicity of sexual contacts in a single evening is just an open invitation to germs to have a ball (if you'll pardon the expression). When I worked regularly at a London VD clinic, I used to see men who had . . .er . . . 'embraced' 25 ladies the previous Saturday night – and who now had to telephone these 25 ladies (and their husbands) to tell them that they urgently needed to go to a clinic for a check-up.

Quite seriously, outbreaks of thrush, gonorrhoea and NSU, of jealousy and even of violence have forced the activities of many wife-swapping circles to grind – so to speak – to a halt.

If AIDS gets a hold among the devotees of wife-swapping orgies (as it has among the *gay* orgy set), then the results could be monumentally disastrous.

Impotence

Let's be quite clear that virtually every man has difficulty in 'making it' at some time in his life. Occasional episodes of this sort are nothing to worry about, and the important thing is that both partners should just do their best not to make a big deal of it!

But it's a different situation when a man keeps on and on having trouble with his potency. This can sap his confidence and ruin his relationship with his partner.

Now why does impotence occur? It's usual to say that some cases are physical, but that most are emotional in origin. But – as a leading article in the *British Medical Journal* recently pointed out – in many men, it is a mixture of the two.

For example, there may be a slight physical problem which sometimes makes it difficult for a man to get a good erection. But he reacts to this with panic and (let's say) his wife reacts to it with scorn, then – bingo – there's now an enormous emotional problem as well.

The average bloke finds it difficult to see how his emotions can make him impotent. But to understand, this we have to look at the mechanisms which cause erection in the human male. I'm sorry to say that these are not completely understood by us docs yet, but broadly speaking, what we do know is this.

Erection happens when blood is suddenly pumped into cavities inside the man's penis. Some sort of valve mechanism seems to stop the blood from flowing out again while he remains sexually excited.

But what causes these extraordinary hydraulic changes in a chap's John Thomas? Basically, they're caused by impulses which flow along the nerves which control the penile blood vessels.

One powerful set of impulses is generated if you stroke your man's penis. This simple action should fire off a spinal reflex which tells the blood vessels to start pumping blood into his male organ.

Another powerful set originates in his brain. If he starts thinking about you in a sexy way, this should send signals down his spine, and into the nerves which lead to the penile blood vessels.

Unfortunately, the chemical mechanism by which all these impulses are sent to his penis is incredibly complex and delicate. And nervousness, tension, depression and even tiredness can block them.

So that's why the emotions play an important part in impotence.

However, there can be physical factors too. Alcohol is the most common of these. Other drugs can also play a part – and these include several of the pills which are widely used for treating high blood pressure. Abuse of 'hard' drugs is also a notorious cause of impotence. While a man's on heroin or cocaine, for example, he's very likely to find he's off the boil sexually.

Actually physical diseases don't commonly cause impotence. But erection difficulties are variously associated with diabetes, disorders of the nerve tissues and with 'hardening of the arteries'.

Hormone deficiencies rarely cause impotence. But being *fat* increases the chances – and slimming down may sometimes put things right.

What all this adds up to I'm afraid, is that there isn't often a simple and easy answer to the problem of impotence. I wish there were a pill which would immediately cure the millions of blokes who are impotent – but there isn't at the moment.

However, a distinguished woman doctor at the Hammersmith Hospital is working on a chemical which might lead to a 'potency pill'.

But in the meantime, what can be done if your fella is impotent? Get him to see a doc, in order to rule out the above-mentioned physical causes. A brief physical examination, plus a couple of blood tests, should be sufficient to sort this out.

Almost invariably, you're then left to face the fact that the problem is basically an emotional one. This is nothing for either of you to be ashamed of. In today's crazy, stress-ridden world, it's not surprising that so many men are too tense, too anxious, too tired or too unhappy to make love!

It's terribly important that you – as his loving partner – should do your best to make him feel both relaxed and wanted at bed-time. Whether he recovers will depend greatly on how much *you* can build up his (probably rather shaken) self-esteem.

Probably the most successful therapists where impotence is concerned are the *behaviourists*, and especially those who practice the famous 'Masters and Johnson' method of therapy. This mainly involves in-depth counselling followed by the 'forbidding' of attempts at intercourse, plus encouragement of non-demanding physical activity between the couple, in a relaxed atmosphere. Dotty though it sounds, this does take 'pressure to perform' off the man – and in an encouraging number of cases, it leads to restoration of potency.

I want to conclude by telling you about one or two slightly more dramatic remedies, some of which offer considerable hope for the future.

However, I do want to emphasise that some of these methods of treatment are still largely experimental. And the results which they can achieve are pretty uncertain.

However, there is one well-tried, low-risk method. It's called 'desensitisation therapy', and it's particularly useful for men whose impotence is caused by anxiety. (Nervousness just at the moment of attempting penetration is a very common cause of sudden collapse of a gent's erection.)

Desensitisation therapy works thus. The man lies on a couch while his therapist encourages him to fantasise about the moment of penetration.

As his nervousness rises, the therapist uses techniques based on pyschotherpay to help him relax. The therapist may even inject small doses of a sedative drug into a vein as the patient reports that his anxiety is increasing. This 'titration of tranquillisation against anxiety' can sometimes be quite helpful in helping a chap overcome the nerves which have been undermining his potency.

Much more drastic is the new technique of injecting certain drugs directly into the penis when you want to have intercourse.

This is still very controversial, but some good results have been reported after injecting with alpha-symphathetic blockers – drugs which affect the nerves which control erection.

But there can be problems. The injection can produce a very prolonged and painful erection, which simply won't go dowm. This can be dangerous.

Also, it's not really practical to keep a doctor in the bedroom to give you a jab in the penis whenever you want to make love. A few specialists have got round this problem by training the man's partner to give the intrapenile injection – but a jab wrongly-aimed by an amateur can be very risky. (I must say, the introduction of this therapy does lend new meaning to the phrase 'Just a little prick . . . ')

Finally, it's sometimes possible for a surgeon to insert a splint. Nowadays this can be inflatable, pumped up when needed.

Q I don't really mind, but I've just discovered that my husband had a 'massage' while away on business in Hong Kong. Is this sort of thing common?

A I'm afraid so, ma'am. Your letter seems to indicate that you've decided to forgive him – and I hope he appreciates that fact.

I do feel sorry for the wife (above) who discovered that her husband had a quick 'massage' while on a business trip to 'Ong Kong. Most women are probably quite unaware that nowadays businessmen and other male travellers constantly have this temptation put in front of them (so to speak).

There are very few major cities you can go to without encountering ads for massage services. Very often, they're a prominent feature of the brochures which are left in your hotel room.

One can't exactly approve of this sort of thing, but I suppose it is at least preferable to prostitution, with its terrible attendant dangers of VD and other infections (not to mention the appalling risk of pregnancy of unknown-origin for the prostitute).

Anyway, I'm fascinated to note that in the massage area too, equality of the sexes is creeping in. Yes:one or two London magazines are now actually carrying ads in which gents offer 'visiting massage' to women.

> LADIES ONLY. Visiting massage service. Tuesday, Wednesday and Thursday only. Des will relax you.

Eager to investigate this new anti-sexist trend, I asked a lady colleague to reply to one of these small ads (*not* the one above). She received a very nice letter from a chap called Leon – who is apparently only too willing to provide tired businesswomen with relaxing body massage.

I'm glad to say that my female colleague didn't take him up on his offer – but she was impressed by the fact that Leon is so devoted to his work that he provides his visiting service free of charge!

Infidelity

Unfortunately, we have to face the fact that infidelity is very common. Various US and British surveys have suggested that as many as 50% of all husbands are unfaithful to their wives at some time.

And recent surveys in the USA and Britain have now confirmed that infidelity is alarmingly common in women too. For instance, studies carried out on the readers of what are generally thought of a highly respectable and conservative women's magazines indicate that at least three out of 10 wives have been unfaithful.

These studies are open to one major criticism, and it's this: women who have very strict and puritanical moral views *tend to refuse to take part in such surveys,* whereas women who are very 'easy-going' sexually are likely to have few inhibitions about answering the questions. So this factor may, of course, artificially inflate the apparent proportion of wives who have been unfaithful to their partners.

Nonetheless, any doctor or marriage guidance counsellor will tell you that it's very common to have to cope with a person who's terribly distraught because he or she has found out about his or her partner's infidelity.

This section isn't about adultery. It's about *how to cope with your partner's adultery.*

So how *are* you going to cope with it? Well, the old ways of 'coping' with infidelity was to set about divorcing your partner immediately – or possibly to make arrangements for shooting them.

That really doesn't seem awfully sensible these days. If *everyone* divorced (or, indeed, shot) his or her spouse solely because of infidelity, there wouldn't be that many marriages left (and rather a lot of bodies around, too).

There's no doubt that finding out that your partner has been unfaithful can be a very shattering experience. Unless you're running some sort of 'open-marriage' you're likely to be extremely upset – to say the least.

In the past, I've seen quite a few women and men who've simply never recovered from the shock of their spouse's infidelity: many years later, they're still depressed and resentful.

But, if you're going to make a go of your marriage, then clearly you have to try and react in a more positive way than this, difficult though it may be.

Here are a few basic suggestions as to how you might deal with the situation:

although it may be terribly hard, try to be generous-minded; have a blazing row if you wish, but always keep in your mind the possibility of forgiveness

think coolly and clearly about just how common such silly affairs are

once you've vented your feelings, try to think about the *temptations* which have made your partner go astray. (Was it during a business trip abroad by one of you? Was she or he lonely and fed up when sudden and seductive 'consolation' – in the shape of sex – was offered?)

painful though it may be, try to think about what *you* have done which might have pushed your partner towards infidelity. (If you don't think you've ever done anything like that, you must indeed be a remarkable and saintly person!)

think particularly about whether you've been tender and loving enough recently

think about whether you've been understanding and sympathetic, and whether you've listened to your partner's problems and worries and tried to help her or him

think about whether you've made yourself *attractive* enough to your partner lately – banal though it sounds, the fact is that again and again, people go off and have sex with somebody else because their own partner has let her – or himself go. I wish I had £10 for every time I've heard a really unwashed and scruffy-looking person saying 'I just can't understand why she/he did it . . .'

finally, think about whether you've taken the trouble to be *sexually pleasing* enough to your partner recently. Again, that sounds trite: yet time and again, wives take lovers because their husbands won't make love to them often enough; or husbands go with other women because their wives aren't sexually adventurous enough in bed.

I know that what I've said will irritate many people, because it puts so much responsibility on the *innocent* party. But if you want to keep the marriage going, then clearly *both* of you (not just the guilty party) have got to work hard at it.

Two final 'no-nos': firstly, don't respond to your partner's infidelity by confessing some past unfaithfulness of your own (if you've had one) – still less by flinging it in his or her face!

Why not? Studies indicate that human beings (i.e. people like your partner) are so idiotic that they tend to regard their own infidelities as 'not very important' – but they tend to regard their spouse's affairs as 'very serious indeed'!

So resist the urge to shriek 'Well – *now* I can tell you that you're not the only one: I did it with the Head Buyer at the office Christmas party!' This won't get you anywhere at all, and it may put another nail in the coffin of the marriage.

Secondly *don't*, if you can avoid it, react to your partner's infidelity by refusing point blank to make love ever again. It's quite natural to want to refuse to make love with someone who's just let you down. On the other hand you have to remember that love (*including* physical love) is exactly what's needed to 're-cement' your marriage.

Refusing to have sex after things have calmed down might just drive your spouse away for good. Remember that you may well now have competition from 'the other woman' or 'the other man' (in a few cases, from both!).

You need to fight this with all the weapons at your command if you want to retain your spouse. And those include your sexual weapons . . .

Good luck – and I hope you keep your relationship together.

Intercourse – Difficulties In

Sexual problems are extremely common, and it is quite obvious that the physical side of many marriages is unsatisfactory to one partner or both. The situation does seem to be improving, however, and this undoubtedly because people in general are today far less ignorant about love-making than they were 20 or even 10 years ago.

Where a husband and wife have difficulties with intercourse, the best thing is if they both sit down and read a good marriage manual, which can be obtained from places like the Family Planning Association (phone number below) or 'Relate' the National Marriage Guidance Council (01-580 1087). Do choose a recent one, however – many of the books which were written a few years back contain all sorts of dangerous myths and misleading information!

A small (but slowly increasing) number of doctors are now undertaking training in the treatment of sexual problems. If your own doctor can't help you, ask him to refer you to someone who can. If in difficulty, ring the Family Planning Information Service on 01-636 7866.

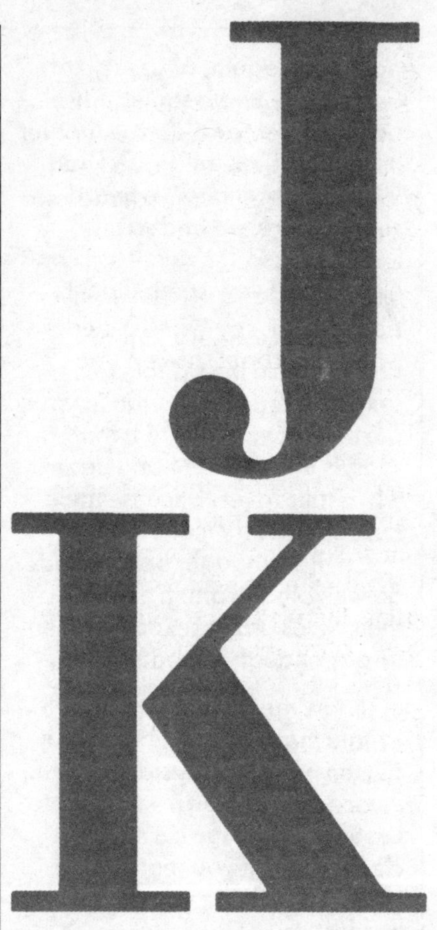

Q We are a husband and wife in the West Country, writing you a joint letter about a serious problem which has soured our marriage. It is jealousy.

(The husband writes:) Every time I go out, my wife is intensely suspicious about how I feel towards other women. She fears that I will become sexually aroused at the sight of them, becomes acutely depressed and can't sleep. In fact, I don't chat up other women or anything like that.

(The wife writes:) Wherever he goes, there's bound to be at least one attractive woman, about whom he might have thoughts. I see this as mental unfaithfulness. It has got to the stage now that whenever he returns home I have to ask if he has been attracted to someone else.

A Your marriage is heading for disaster unless you do something about it. The most encouraging thing is you've written me a JOINT letter – which does suggest that both of you want to work your way to a solution.

All normal people feel some degree of jealousy over the person they love. (Indeed, when jealousy vanishes, that's often an indication that love has gone.) But in this case, the jealousy has really reached the stage of an obsessional neurosis. In other words, you're now ill. To save your health and your marriage, ask your GP to refer you for psychotherapy immediately.

Having read your husband's contribution to your anguished joint letter, I'm sure he loves you and will help and support you. Good luck to you both.

Q Recently, I was very surprised to find that I was willing to go to bed with a guy and have intercourse, but then discovered that I was really a bit repelled by the idea of having him kiss me. Do you think I am abnormal?

A Nope. For a lot of women, a kiss seems to be more intimate than sexual intercourse.

I'd guess that you weren't very interested in this bloke, this is probably a good indication that you shouldn't waste your time going to bed with him again.

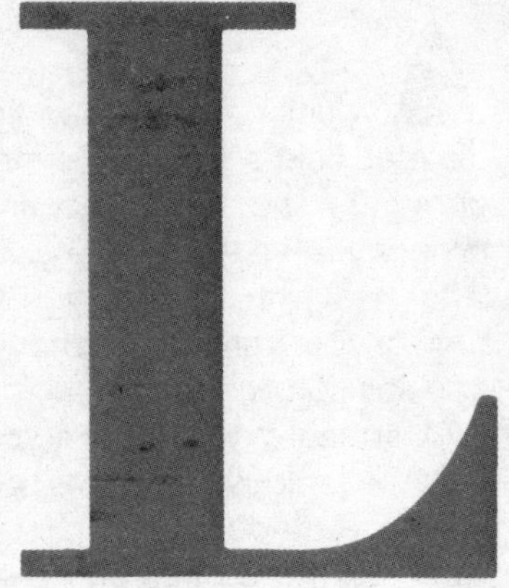

Q My wife and I were engaged in love play the other night when she admitted to me that when she was at university, she'd had a lesbian relationship with a woman who is now one of our best friends. This relevation turned me on at the time, but I'm a bit worried. Do you think my wife might be basically homosexual?

A I really doubt if your missus will turn out to be one of what are sometimes called 'Les Girls'. You see, it is fantastically common in young women to have brief physical relationships with each other, particularly when they're lonely and away from home. When you consider how readily younger women snuggle up to one another and how quite cheerfully they share beds (in a way that would be anathema to most of us chaps!), it's scarcely surprising that they sometimes 'slide over the border' into sexual contact.

As a matter of fact, the amazing Dr Kinsey found that no less than 30% of young college girls had had a physical relationship with another woman. Many of them were probably homesick and need of a cuddle, like your wife perhaps.

To give you a f'rinstance of how common this kind of thing is, even one of Britain's best-known agony columnists is perfectly open about having had two youthful homosexual relationships. (And in case anybody's wondering – no, it *isn't* me!).

Q I wonder if you can answer a very difficult question for me?

Why is my husband admitting that he occasionally gets turned on by the idea of lesbianism?

A Can't tell you for certain, but there's no doubt that – bizarrely enough – vast numbers of gents seem to be intrigued by the idea of women caressing each other.

Studies of men's secret fantasies have shown this quite clearly. Furthermore, I am told that both orgies and live 'sex shows' usually feature girl-to-girl lovemaking in an attempt to excite the male audience.

This is really all a bit baffling, isn't it? After all, you don't find women going around proclaiming to be turned on by the idea of guys going in for homosexual lovemaking. (At least, I don't think so anyway.)

Q I am a widow, and after many years of lusty heterosexual life with my late husband. I am amazed to find that I've fallen into an occasional warm lesbian relationship with a dear friend. Is this illegal?

A No ma'am. Oddly enough, lesbian love-making (unlike male homosexual activity) has never been illegal in Britain. It's claimed that this is because of the fact that when the appropriate law was due to be passed in the 19th century, no one had the nerve to explain it to Queen Victoria.

Q I was very upset to learn that my daughter – age 21 – is regularly sleeping with her boyfriend at the weekends. Is there any way I can stop them?

A I fear not, ma'am. I understand how you feel – but life has changed, and the fact is that most young adult women go to bed with their boyfriends these days.

Indeed, a recent survey showed that over a third of under-25s do lead a decidedly more promiscuous life than that – with three or more partners a year. Be grateful that your daughter isn't apparently one of this group, but just has one steady (and, I hope, loving) male friend.

Living Together

One of the amazing changes of recent years has been the vast increase in the habit of living together. Twenty years ago, you couldn't publicly admit that you were living together: yet nowadays, every other pop star seems to have a 'live-in-lover' – and a very high proportion of young adults are doing the same thing.

In some instances there is a definite case for living together. When I survey the shattered marriages of people who only managed to make it through the first three or four months of matrimony (and then found out they couldn't *stand* one another!), I seriously wonder why they didn't avoid all the trouble and legal complications by living together on a trial basis first.

I note that there is one world-famous female media pundit whose views on marriage are avidly quoted in newspapers and TV. *Her* only marriage lasted three weeks! Why couldn't she just have moved in with the man for a month or two, discovered they were incompatible, and saved the vicar all that trouble for nothing?

Also, there is a widespread feeling today that living together is at least 'stable' and therefore preferable to the promiscuity which so many young adults adopt. On the other hand, there are difficulties and dangers in the 'living-together' relationship. They can be summed up briefly like this:

parents and relatives may still be very upset

you need to be very clear about what happens if somebody gets pregnant – which they frequently do. (If it happens, *don't* rush into matrimony just to 'give the baby a name' – a hurried marriage is *never* a good idea.)

sordid and commercial though it sounds, you've also got to be very clear about what your *financial* arrangements are going to be – regrettably, many live-in couples run into all sorts of bitter financial disputes when they break up. It's a pretty awful business when two former lovers meet up in court to fight over who gets half the house or – in the USA – who pays 'palimony'.

So, think twice before you accept that tempting invitation to 'move in with me, darling!' You could be letting yourself in for a lot of happiness – or for a lot of trouble.

Q **My live-in boyfriend is a great guy and a wonderful lover. But he seems to have one problem that I'm too embarrassed to ask him about.**

Every time he goes for a pee in the night, he misses the toilet. As a result, there is usually a slight puddle for me to clear up.

Do you think there's anything wrong with him?

A Nope – except he should be clearing up his own 'puddles'.

I must admit that there's a chance that he might have a moderately common anatomical abnormality of the penis (present in about one man in 200), which makes it a bit difficult to avoid peeing on the floor.

But another explanation is much likelier.

When a bloke has been sexually excited, his 'love juices' (as us doctors call them) tend to create a slight blockage in the urinary pipe for a little while.

This makes it very difficult for the gent to 'aim straight' when he next visits the loo. If you ask your boyfriend, I think he'll confirm that this the cause of the damp patch.

Q **I was engaging in some very enthusiastic love play with my husband last week when he suddenly said to me, 'Ouch! Don't twist so hard, or you'll break it.'**

This quite alarmed me! Is it really possible for a woman to break a man's penis, in the same way that one can break a wrist or an arm?

A Yes, ma'am – this is a risk that all energetic ladies should know about.

Although your husband's penis doesn't have a bone in it (at least not unless he's a badger or something), it does become almost as stiff as bone when he's excited. This is because it's absolutely packed to bursting point with blood.

The blood is contained in three cylinders (each about the size of a panatella cigar) which run the length of his 'John Thomas'.

If you unwisely grasp his erect organ and twist it violently to one side, you can cause an extremely painful fracture of one or more of these cylinders.

This is a genuine surgical emergency if it occurs, and the unfortunate victim has to be taken to hospital. Usually, his penis is then packed in ice – and he may well have to be taken to theatre to have the blood clot removed from inside it. This is not a lot of fun.

So ladies – whatever you do to your gents in bed, PLEASE eschew all forms of violent twisting manipulation!

However, bear in mind that the secret information which I have imparted to you today can be used as a defence against rapists.

If you are ever attacked by a naked man with an erect penis, simply grasp it as firmly as you can – and forcibly rearrange it from 12 o'clock to six o'clock – and then run like hell.

Q My fiancée has just started using a peppermint 'body lotion' during lovemaking. When it gets into her vagina, it gives us both quite an exciting sensation. But is it safe to use it like this?

A It's quite well-known that peppermint-flavoured lotions do give both partners an agreeable tingle.

However, introducing chemicals and flavourings into the vagina can cause a sensitivity reaction, in which the delicate tissues (yours too) become sore and red. So I reckon that your fiancée should be a little wary about what she puts into her vagina. Come to think of it, that's not a bad maxim for all women everywhere . . .

Q What worries me is this: since so many men have slightly dirty or scruffy fingernails, couldn't vaginal love play lead to infection?

A Yup – you're right. Digital stimulation of the inside of the vagina is the second commonest form of male-female love play. It is most frequently done with the middle finger.

Now simple inspection of a series of men's hands will quickly demonstrate that not all of their fingernails are 100% clean. (Indeed, at the end of a long working day, this would be bacteriologically impossible.)

So transfer of germs to the vagina does happen – and it's possible that those germs might lead to a vaginal discharge. However, the types of germs found on the fingers aren't usually the same ones which cause a discharge (which is good news).

On the other hand (so to speak) there could also be an association between dirty finger nails and cancer of the cervix. You see, I've been pointing out for years that male manual occupations are linked with a higher risk of cervical cancer in the female partner.

This is possibly because men who do manual work are more likely to bring home dirt in their fingernails.

So the moral is fairly clear. I don't want to stop anybody's bedtime fun – or to deprive women of a very useful source of sexual fulfilment – but gentlemen readers: do please make sure that anything you put inside a woman is clean! (And I do mean *anything*...).

Why Love play?

Yes, why have love play? What's the point of it all?

Quite a few bewildered people (mostly of the male persuasion) ask that question. They can't quite see why sex needs to be more than a question of a man putting his penis inside a woman and thrusting away like mad – just like they do in the men's magazines.

But in the real world, things aren't like that at all! For a start, one thing that every young lad needs to know is that most women will not have a climax unless they are given a little love play – certainly before intercourse, perhaps during it, and possibly afterwards too.

Strange as it may seem, this comes as shattering news to many males. But it's true. The majority of women don't usually reach a climax during intercourse itself – only during love play. So for them, no love play usually means no climax (and, almost certainly, no *multiple* climaxes). Furthermore, every man needs to know that nearly all women find intercourse uncomfortable or even downright painful *if there hasn't been preliminary love play*.

Why? Firstly because love play makes the woman's vagina start secreting those famous 'love juices' which are so absolutely vital to lubricate the process of intercourse. Without them, the vagina would be so dry that intercourse would be very unpleasant indeed for the woman (and not a lot of fun for most men).

Secondly, preliminary love play makes the vaginal muscles — which guard the opening of the vagina — open up in preparation to receive the penis. If a man tries to enter before that initial opening up process is completed, the woman will feel discomfort and even pain. And in the case of some couples, he won't be able to get in at all – this is a common cause of non-consummation of a marriage!

Thirdly, love play makes the woman's vagina lengthen as she gets more sexually excited – so that there is much more room inside.

But, dear female readers: you aren't the only ones who need love play. Your partner will benefit greatly from it too.

Why? Well, once again let's look at the purely mechanical aspect of sex for a moment. Vast numbers of men have difficulties and worries over their erections. 'Will I be able to get it hard? . . . 'Will it *stay* hard? . . . 'Will it collapse on me?'

That's one reason why so many of them do stupid things like leap inside a woman the moment they've achieved an erection – they're terrified it might collapse!

But if man's in bed with a woman who is skilled at love play, he need have no anxieties whatever. For with deft fingers and lips, she will assuredly bring him to an erection – perhaps many times in an evening, depending how matters develop.

Indeed, I'm convinced that a woman who is really adept at love play could cure most cases of impotence single-handed (so to speak). Would that there were more such women around!

Actually, even the most active and 'virile' of males who has no doubts or anxieties about his 'performance' will nonetheless benefit from being on the receiving end of skilled love play techniques. This is partly because love play plays such an important role in romance but the other point to make about love play is this. *It's so very nice!*

Romance and Love Play

One of the main reasons that love play is so good is that is awfully romantic! Yes, romantic. Love play is of course the natural progression of, say, a candlelit dinner, with soft lights, sweet music and the gentle touch of the hands across the dining table. Without love play, there can be no romance.

Consider the sort of awful situations in which there is a complete *absence* of love play, and you will see that they represent the exact opposite of romance. Here are a few such situations:

a man going with a prostitute for a five-minute encounter

a man coming home drunk and forcing himself on his wife

a woman being raped

In all of these unpleasant situations, the contact between man and woman is basic, squalid and brutish. There's no romance – and, of course, there's no love play.

How very different when two people love each other and want to make each other happy! Right from the start, they do everything they can to 'pleasure' one another – and to make each other feel good and warm and wanted. In short, they use love play – which is an essential ingredient of any romantic relationship between a man and a woman.

General Caressing

How does love play begin? Well, as you can see from the title of this section, it usually begins with General Caressing. And a fine old soldier he was too . . .

I use the word 'general' because it is very important that the man – in particular – should always take care to avoid starting with any kind of *direct* approach to the woman's genitals.

Many males don't realize that most females are very definitely turned off by sudden, premature, unsubtle approaches to the vaginal region. Some men hold the touching belief that if you make a quick lunge towards a woman's vagina, she will promptly melt into your arms – but that is, of course, nonsense.

No: what nearly all women prefer is an indirect (and – yes! – romantic) approach in which the man:

says nice things and tells her he loves her

strokes her hair

holds her hand

strokes her shoulders

strokes her arms

strokes her back

All of these actions, you'll notice, are pleasant and arousing – but sexually non–demanding. If a man does them to a woman, she can enjoy them without feeling pressurized. (This was really one of the great discoveries that the old firm of Masters and Johnson made in their researches at their sex clinic in St Louis, Missouri: they found that non-sexual caressing was a great way of building up somebody's confidence and making them feel relaxed and happy.

From this stage, the experienced lover will move on to rather more specifically sexual caresses – but, if he's wise, without yet making a direct approach to the woman's vagina.

For example, he can:

caress her buttocks

stroke her legs

fondle her breasts

and, of course, kiss these parts of her body too.

Research with the amazing vaginal probe at London's Institute of Psychiatry shows very clearly that while this sort of pleasant caressing is going on, a woman's vagina does start preparing itself for love-making as she becomes more and more aroused.

Much the same principles of gradually increasing stimulation apply if you are a woman caressing your man. However, I have to admit that most men do prefer a rather more direct approach than is favoured by most women. So very few males will complain if a female fairly rapidly starts transferring her attention to his penis. Now read on . . .

Love play with the Fingers

So let's now move on to actual love-play with the fingers – what many people call 'petting'. A lot of people get very embarrassed about this subject, and think that there is something terribly 'rude' about using your fingers to give your loved one sexual pleasure. But in actual fact, it's very hard to see how a couple could have a really good and satisfying sexual relationship if they didn't go in for 'finger-play'. Certainly, very few women would reach orgasm without it. (And still fewer would reach multiple orgasms.)

However, love-play with the fingers is *not* an instinctive thing: you have to know what to do. If you do *not* know what to do, you will hurt your partner!

This is actually very common – especially among newly-weds. The couple leap into bed and, before very long, she makes a lunge for his penis and gives it a rather violent tweak. Result: he doubles up in temporary agony!

More seriously, a man can do a woman quite a lot of harm with clumsy, unskilled attempts at finger petting. What often happens is that he cuts her – externally or internally – with his fingernails. This can cause pain, and quite a lot of bleeding. And, most importantly, the pain may put her off sex for a very long time – and indeed help to cause the common sex difficulty called 'vaginismus'. So, when using finger-play:

- be sure your nails aren't jagged
- be gentle
- if necessary, use a lubricant
- make sure you know what you're doing – and
- practise!

Now, what exactly do you do! Let us look first at the nice things a man can do for a woman – and then at the equally nice things she can do to him.

Things Men Can Do for Women

OK, so you're going to use your fingertips to give your partner pleasure. Begin by *gently* brushing your fingertips past the opening of her vagina. *Don't* rush things, and don't do anything silly like trying to ram a finger straight in immediately.

Instead, lovingly stroke the outside of her vagina. If you've wooed her carefully, lovingly and romantically, you'll find that she's already beginning to become moist with love juices.

Next, use the pads of your fingers to caress the area of her clitoris. Rub gently on either side of it – or, if she prefers it, rub directly on it (though not all women like this). *Ask her what she likes*. There's no point in lying there doing something that simply doesn't turn her on!

If things are very dry round her clitoris, it may be worthwhile scooping up a little of her love juice on your fingertips. But if there's not much of it around, then there is no reason why you shouldn't lick your fingertips.

Alternatively, some couples use a lubricant, such as baby oil – or one of the lubricants sold in sex shops.

Learning how to stimulate a woman's clitoris properly is one of the great loving arts, which every man should master – though remarkably few do. If in doubt, remember: keep it gentle, but *fast*. And do what she likes – not what *you* think is best!

Once she is really moist, you may well wish to move on to the next stage of finger-play, which is slipping a finger *inside* her vagina. That is a very good preparation for intercourse; if more bridegrooms knew how to do it, there'd be fewer unconsummated marriages.

You can use any of your fingers, but the middle one is usually the most effective. Slide it in gently.

Then move it gently but rapidly

in and out. Do *not* make the movements too vigorous, or you may catch her delicate tissues with your fingernail. If you follow this finger technique properly, you'll find that your thumb or forefinger will, at the same time rub gently against the region of her clitoris – so giving her added stimulation.

I'm not exaggerating when I say that really *mastering* this technique may take you years. Yet mastering it will pay rich dividends, in terms of the pleasure and satisfaction you'll give to your loved one.

But once you are reasonably adept at the 'middle finger method', then you can try some of the following:

put your thumb inside instead, and gently rotate it

put your middle *and* index fingers in, and use the pads of the two fingertips gently to stimulate her G-spot

use your index finger to stimulate the sensitive *sides* of her vagina

use a finger pad to stimulate the back wall of her vagina (though not all women like this, so be guided by what the lady tells you)

use the tips of two fingers to stimulate her cervix gently

At all times, be gentle and sensitive. Take your lead from the speed and intensity of her breathing, from any little moans of pleasure she makes – and, above all, from what she asks you to do!

Things Women Can Do for Men

Now what can a woman do with her fingers to please a man?

Well, we men don't have as many (or as interesting) sex organs as you do. But we do have several areas which are very sensitive to soft female fingertips.

First of all, you can stroke your partner's nipples – most men like this. You will find that his nipple gets a little erection, though not on the same scale as yours.

Next, you can stroke his testicles. This will not bring a man to a climax, but it's an agreeable and sometimes rather comforting sensation for him.

And finally, of course, there's his penis. There are various ways of stimulating this with your fingers. In practice, you need to find out what the man you love likes having done to his organ.

So for heaven's sake, ask him! Half the mix-ups and confusions in people's beds are caused by the fact that so many couples are too embarrassed to speak while they're trying to get each other excited.

It's not generally known that you may well find it easier to do this sort of love-play if you actually anoint his penis with a little baby oil, or other bland lubricant. I gather that some men prefer talcum powder.

You may also find it helpful to hold his testicles with your other hand while you are gently rubbing his penis. Girls in massage parlours (who, I assume, probably know more about this than most people) have a technique in which they increase pleasurable tension in the penis by holding the testicles downwards with one hand while they rub the male organ with the other.

All these finger techniques are useful in adding fun and fulfilment to a loving relationship. Don't worry – as some women do – that you will damage your partner's penis by handling it. (Remember, you're far more likely to damage his ego by *not* handling it.)

However, in a vigorous session of love play, you should take care not to do two things when it's erect:

don't twist it violently to one side – this is an occasional cause of quite serious injury (it's also quite a good thing to do to a would-be rapist!)

don't 'twang' it back violently towards his feet – when it's erect, it's *not* meant to go that way.

Love play with the Lips and Tongue

Naturally, the mouth plays a very important part in love play. Kissing your partner all over is immensely agreeable – as is being kissed all over in return.

When you are doing this, you can of course combine caressing with your tongue. And don't forget those little nibbles and 'love-bites', which most people like being on the receiving end of.

But . . . it's best not to go in for love-bites around the sexual parts of the body, where they may cause damage and excessive pain.

What about love-biting the breasts? Some women like this, others don't – and may even be frightened by it. It's probably best not to love-bite the nipples (which are very sensitive in both sexes) but just to confine yourself to gentle sucking.

Now to the controversial subject of kissing the 'naughty bits'. I don't know why people still get so het up about this subject, but a lot of them are offended by it, even today.

In fact, kissing someone in their most intimate part is the most natural and delightful way of showing your love – and of giving him or her great pleasure. It's certainly not to everybody's taste, but research does indicate that the majority of younger couples now go in for it.

Mouth-play for a Man to Use on a Woman

So how can a man pleasure the woman he loves by using his lips and tongue? It's really quite simple. If you're a man who isn't used to this sort of thing, then just begin by giving long, lingering kisses to the upper part of your partner's pubic hair.

From there, you can move down and gently kiss the region of her clitoris. This gives most women tremendous pleasure and satisfaction – and it's a very useful way of helping the woman who has difficulty in reaching a climax.

Next you can gently titillate her clitoris with the tip of your tongue. This isn't easy to begin with, but after a little practice you'll find it tremendously effective in pleasing her.

Finally, there's a technique which gives many women great pleasure, but which not all men are keen on trying. It involves actually putting the tongue inside her vagina.

It's certainly well worth having a go at, though it's like oysters – a bit of an acquired taste! All you do is gently insert your tongue into your partner's vagina, and gently move it in and out. This is very effective – though if the lady gets very enthusiastic, you may find it a trifle difficult to draw breath!

Mouth-play for a Woman to Use on a Man

Now, what nice things can a woman do for her partner with her mouth? Basically it's just a question of using your lips and tongue to give him pleasure. You can, if you wish, take one of his testicles in your mouth – be very gentle since they are rather sensitive!

You can also kiss the area of skin just *behind* his testicles – an area which is very sexually receptive in most males.

But the thing which men appreciate most is direct stimulation of the penis. You can do this in three ways:

simply kissing it (a nice, loving thing to do)

licking it with your tongue (this is very sexually stimulating – and a great help to the man who has difficulty getting an erection)

putting it in your mouth and sucking (be careful not to give him a painful jab with your teeth!)

Once again, oral love-play techniques on the penis (termed 'fellatio') aren't to *everybody's* taste. But research shows that a very high proportion of couples do now enjoy it.

Incidentally, you'll find that these oral love play techniques on your partner are often best performed while he's doing much the same thing to you. This involves taking up the famous '69' or '*soixante-neuf*' position, in which the couple's bodies roughly resemble the figure '69' on the bed.

Putting Things in the Vagina

Be very cautious about putting anything in the vagina except what nature intended for it! Unfortunately, some of those frightful and tacky men's magazines at the cheaper end of the market have given a lot of young males the notion that it's a good idea to play silly games with cucumbers, bananas and whatnot. This no way to get your vitamin C!

Seriously, foreign bodies might possibly carry infection. *Hard* foreign bodies can damage the vagina – I have certainly encountered one case in which terrible damage was done to a woman because her husband was stupid enough to put a wooden rod inside.

And most hospital casualty officers are familiar with those incredible cases in which a woman arrives in an ambulance with a bottle or a jar jammed inside her. It's all right to put a clean vibrator in the vagina if you want to do so, but no other objects.

Incidentally, words fail me at the idea given world-wide prominence in Shirley Conran's novel *Lace* – that a man can give a woman pleasure by putting a *goldfish* inside her vagina. If I heard of anybody doing such a stupid thing, I'd report them to the RSPCA (and that isn't a joke!)

Rectal Love Play or 'Bottom-play'

This seems to be almost universal among sophisticated couples these days (partly as a result of the influence of Marlon Brando's film *Last Tango in Paris*). I suppose it's not altogether surprising, since nature for some reason has equipped the bottom with a lot of sexually excitable nerve endings.

Rather astonishingly, there's no doubt that many women can reach a climax simply through having the rectal opening gently stimulated with a fingertip. This activity is called *postillionage*.

Also, as readers of Harold Robbins novels will know, it's quite easy for a woman to slip a well-lubricated finger up a man's bottom and massage his prostate gland. This definitely helps some men get aroused, and gives an intense and rather unusual climax.

But . . . what the films and novels don't make clear is that the back passage is, of course, a germ-laden area of the body. To be blunt, a finger placed there will come away with germs on it. As you probably know there's now not the slightest doubt that the germ of AIDS can be transmitted by the rectal activities of homosexual blokes.

I'm not suggesting that tickling your loved one's backside will give you AIDS. But if you decide to go in for this sort of thing, then at the very least you ought to wash your hand afterwards. On no account put it near her/his genitals (or your own) till this has been done.

Incidentally, bottom-play without a lubricant is likely to be *very* uncomfortable, and may cause bleeding. This is why sales of butter are alleged to have gone up so dramatically after the aforementioned Marlon Brando film.

Using Drugs to Heighten Love play

This is widespread – and absolutely mad. I cannot overemphasize the fact that drugs like heroin, cocaine and the various substances that people 'sniff' are likely to take away your sex drive, ruin your health, and very possibly kill you.

Some experts appear to think that *small* amounts of alcohol and 'pot' (which is, of course, illegal in most countries) can safely be used to relax people and so make love play more agreeable. However, any doctor will tell you that *larger* amounts of alcohol have a serious adverse effect on people's love-lives – hence the well-known euphemism for impotence: 'brewer's droop'.

To sum up, don't spoil your love play with drugs. They aren't a passport to instant happiness – in fact, they're more likely to be a passport to the grave.

M

Q **I am a married woman of 40, and my husband is 50. I recently had a short affair with a young man of 20, and was surprised to find that he was able to make love to me much more often than my husband is.**

My husband is only able to have sex once a night. Is there anything he could take to make him more virile?

A No, ma'am. And if your husband is making love once a night at 50, he's doing very well. The average man of 50 does it less than twice a week.

And it's normal for a man of 20 to be able to make love to you much more often than a bloke of 50 can. After all, 20 goes into 40 more often than 50 does . . .

Q **I am much more interested in sex than my husband, so I have to persuade him (verbally and manually) to make love as often as I want to. My worry is this: could I do him any harm by over-stimulating him?**

A No – it's impossible to harm any man or woman by 'over-stimulating' them. The worst that will happen is that he may get a trifle tired.

Q **My husband (aged 35) used to be a very enthusiastic lover, but nowadays he doesn't seem to be interested in making love to me for a second time during an evening. Do you think he's losing his virility?**

A Like many people, you're expecting too much orgasmically of your partner! Many men can only manage it once in an evening. And at 35, the average male has about two orgasms per week. So let the poor bloke rest if he wants to.

Q **My husband – age 40 – can only make love once in an evening. Previous lovers of mine could do it twice. Is he OK?**

A Perfectly OK, ma'am. Unfortunately, many women do tend to overestimate the ability of us chaps to achieve multiple climaxes.

In fact, the ability to make love more than once in an evening depends largely on age.

Research indicates that the percentage of men who regularly (as opposed to occasionally) 'come' more than once in a night is roughly as follows:

Under 16	20%
16–20	15%
21–30	9%
31–40	6%
41–50	2.5%
51–60	3.5%

Q **I had a hysterectomy four months ago, but no one has said anything about making love to my husband again. I feel I am being unfair to him, and I also want to make love. How soon can we?**

A I find it incredible that no one at the hospital had the sense to tell you this. Following most hysterectomies, it's possible to start making love (with care) about six weeks after the op, but always ask your surgeon.

Q **I am a young Asian woman, and I became pregnant as a result of rape. I had a termination, and the man then blackmailed me into having sex with him again. This led to another termination of pregnancy. But I am now free of this man's influence.**

The problem is that my parents have now arranged a marriage for me. Would my bridegroom-to-be be able to tell that I have had two abortions?

A No, he wouldn't. I'm dreadfully sorry to read your appalling story. Quite frankly, it makes my fists itch to thump the bloke who raped and blackmailed you. I think that before you embark on matrimony, you desperately need some personal advice and counselling – eg from the *Brook Advisory Centres For Young People*. Ring their HQ on 01–580 2991. Good luck.

Q I have just got married, and the thing I find most embarrassing about living with a man for the first time is that he is able to hear me pee when I visit the loo, which has a very thin door! How can I cope with this?

A Well ma'am, in the *short* term, you could get a thicker loo door – or just turn the taps on while you're spending a penny. But in the long term, this is one of the things that couples simply have to adjust to. It may take some years before you feel equable about your man overhearing the tinkling noises produced by your bodily functions.

Marriage

Obviously, this book can't be a complete and infallible treatise on marriage. But from the experience of watching a large number of savable marriages break up – mainly because one or both parties persisted in behaving in a way that was silly, immature and selfish – I would suggest these few almost laughably simple ground rules:

when you have problems, *talk* to your partner: 'bottling it up' is likely to lead to disaster

try every day to *praise* your partner – not to criticize him or her

if things are going wrong sexually, *seek professional help* before matters get any worse

try not to commit adultery – it's awfully common, but the troubles it can bring are enormous

if you *do* commit adultery, keep quiet about it; if you must unburden some guilt, find a good friend, doctor, priest or counsellor to talk to, but don't shift the unhappiness onto your poor old spouse

if you suspect or find out that your partner has had an affair, try not to regard it as the end of the marriage

don't seek answers to marriage problems in drink or drugs – a very high proportion of divorces are related to alcohol abuse

don't involve your children in difficulties between you and your spouse – and never try to 'recruit' them onto your side

if the going's get rough, always go and see a trained marriage guidance counsellor ('Relate' is the new name for the Marriage Guidance Council)

try to ensure that your partner is sexually happy: an awful lot of men and women pay no real attention to their spouses' sexual needs – and then wonder why the said spouse goes off with somebody else.

If all that advice sounds a bit trite, I can tell you that I have known quite a few couples who've managed to save their marriages by deciding to stick to rules like these, after a period in which they had been very close to breaking up.

Q My boyfriend has a great body, and is truly fantastic in bed. He would like us to get married. But the big problem is this. Don't think me snobbish, but he comes from a much lower social class than me, and it's not just that, my Mum thinks he's 'awfully rough', and quite unsuitable, darling', the real point is that I am a university graduate, and he is a labourer, and the difference in our IQs must be 40 or 50 points.

A I take it you're telling me that yours is bigger than his?

Seriously, I don't think the difference in your 'social standing' is all that important these days. After all, I've known doctors marry lorry-drivers.

But a 40 or 50-point difference in IQ is another matter. Be warned. This bloke may be a great lover, but if his IQ is 90 and yours is 135, you're not going to have a lot to talk about. That's a classic case of a Radio 3 woman marrying a Radio 1 man.

Q I have had to have a mastectomy. I'm 23, about to be married, and my fiancé honestly accepts me as I am, which is marvellous.

But I cannot think of my body as

attractive, and I feel that other people would be shocked if they know how I looked without clothes.

A I bet you look very nice without clothes – and I'm sure that your fiancé will demonstrate (through his physical love) just how attractive you really are.

Meantime, you need help in building up your confidence, and in dealing with the practical difficulties of having lost a breast. Please contact the splendid *Mastectomy Association*, at *26 Harrison Street, London, WC1H 8JG*.

Q Something very upsetting happened to me recently. First, I should explain that I was widowed at an early age, and have brought up my daughter on my own. She is now a teenager.

I don't have any boyfriends, but I do have sexual feelings, which for a long time I have relieved by masturbation.

A few months ago, I was lying on my bed, relieving my sexual tensions in this way. To my embarrassment, my daugher walked in.

She was terribly shocked. I could not reason with her, and in fact the whole thing has caused a dreadful rift between us. She has

Masturbation

A surprising number of women still think that there's something wrong or shameful about masturbation – and a few still believe that it has harmful effects, like damaging your eyesight!

But I think most people are now aware that masturbation is completely harmless. Survey after survey has shown that the majority of women have masturbated at some time.

Indeed, this widespread knowledge has itself led to a new source of confusion. There are now quite a few women who think they're 'abnormal' because they don't masturbate! Nothing could be further from the truth. Though the sex surveys do show that the vast majority of adult females have masturbated at some time or other, the fact is that a very substantial number *haven't*. And even among those women who *have* gone in for it, there are many for whom it's just a very intermittent sort of pleasure – often amounting to little more than a comforting stroke through the nightdress on a cold winter's evening.

So medically speaking, the point about masturbation is that it's entirely up to you. Whether you do it or not, you're definitely not 'abnormal'. It's true that many sex therapists do now believe that masturbation is a help to a lot of women: as a reliever of tension; as an aid when there's difficulty in reaching orgasm; and even in relieving a period pain. But no one is obliged to do it!

However, just a few words of warning: women (like men) sometimes do rather silly things when masturbating. For instance, a doctor friend of mine treated a young woman who'd done appreciable harm to her vagina by putting an electric toothbrush inside it. Similarly, I've recently had several letters from doctors about patients who have caused injuries to their clitorises by over-violent manipulation with various objects. And there are also occasional cases of women who very unwisely try to masturbate by pushing things like hairgrips in and out of the urinary pipe. This is madness – there's a high risk that the object will vanish up into the bladder!

So if you want to masturbate (and for many women – especially single, divorced or widowed women – it's undoubtedly a pleasant and soothing experience) it's best to stick to gentle rubbing alongside the clitoris, using either a finger or a vibrator, as you prefer!

scarcely spoken to me since then, and is obviously quite disgusted by what she saw.

A This is awfully sad. I'm afraid it's a fact that one generation finds it hard to come to terms with another generation's sexuality – and your poor daughter simply cannot adjust to the idea that you (her Mum) are a sexual being with normal sexual urges.

To begin with, the most important thing you can do is show her all the love and tenderness you can – no matter how she rejects you. If you get cross with her (which would be very understandable), it'll only confirm her bitter opinion of you.

Next, if you can get her talking, it's vital that you try and get over to her that you *still* love her Dad and think fondly of him. She probably worships his memory, and feels that you were being 'unfaithful' to him.

It might be worth saying to her that many men would actually *prefer* their widows to go on feeling sexy. In a way, it's a tribute to the warm love-life that they once shared together.

It would be nice if you could persuade your daughter to go

along with you to one of the *Brook Advisory Centres for Young People* (HQ phone number *01 580 2991*) to have a chat with one of their counsellors – who would, I think, say the same sort of things that I've said here. Good luck.

Q I have a nagging worry about my lover, who is 26. (I am 39.) We've been together for three years, and have a very active sex life, with no inhibitions.

One night we made love several times, and also enjoyed several other forms of sex play.

But the next morning, he told me that during the night he'd woken up feeling very aroused, and couldn't get back to sleep. So he'd gone into the bathroom and mast-urbated.

I can't understand why he needs to do this on his own. It's as if he'd done it in a world of his own that I don't seem to be part of.

A I do understand that you must have felt 'excluded' by the fact that he went off alone in the middle of the night and had a climax.

But the truth is that many people do 'touch themselves up' when their partners are asleep.

Your partner is clearly a young virile guy who needs quite a lot of sex. He obviously didn't want to disturb your sleep – after a hectic evening's love-making – and I think you should concentrate on the fact that he was thoughtful enough and considerate enough *not* to wake you up and demand more sex.

Which – let's face it – is what a heck of a lot of more selfish people would have done!

Q I recently married my second husband, who is aged 53. He is rather unwilling to make love in the mornings (which is my favourite time), unless I first stimulate him manually. Is he im-potent?

A Not at all, ma'am! Like vintage motor cars, many men above a certain age do need to be started by hand – especially on these chilly morns. *Do* warm your hands first, won't you?

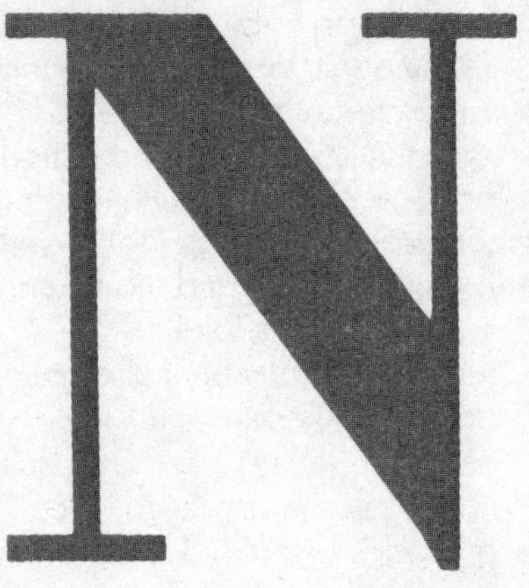

Naughty Underwear

I think it's perfectly reasonable to say that naughty underwear could put a bit of extra fun into a couple's relationship – and perhaps get their love-life going.

The common items are see-through and 'baby-doll' nighties, G-strings, peek-a-boo bras, and open-crotch knickers. For males, there are also *very* abbreviated briefs and 'posing pouches'.

I need hardly say that you don't have to go to a sex shop to get naughty undies. A lot of these items can now be bought quite easily (and possibly considerably cheaper) in high street stores.

Q My fiancé and I were reading your article about lactation when he squeezed his nipple – and out came a little fluid! Why?

A He must have felt a right . . . er . . . wally! Seriously, men do sometimes produce a milky fluid – particularly if their nipples have been stimulated. Some tranquillisers can also make a man secrete a little 'milk'.

Q **My husband wants me to put a couple of gold rings through my nipples. Do you think I should agree to this?**

A I don't think so – unless it's what *you* want to do.

I reckon that there's been a regrettable increase in all this 'body jewellery' nonsense as a result of the publicity surrounding Sally Beauman's best-selling novel *Destiny* – in which a female character is said to wear a diamond in an unusual and extremely uncomfortable place (a place where it would be a *very* serious hazard for any gent who wanted to make love to her!)

Seriously, 'body piercing' in order to insert jewellery into your delicate places does carry quite a risk of causing infection, bleeding, and pain. I wouldn't have anything to do with it if I were you.

The Nipple

The nipple is one of the most sexually sensitive areas of the body – *in both women and men*. Quite a few women can actually reach a climax just through having their nipples stimulated, although I don't know of any males who experience this.

Most people use the word 'nipple' wrongly – they think it means the *whole* of the pigmented disc in the middle of the breast, but it is, in fact, only the central protuberance; the disc which surrounds it is called the areola. The areola is quite sensitive too, but it does not have as many nerve endings as the nipple. The areola may be pink, brown or black – depending on your general colouring. It can be anything up to 12.5 cm (5 ins) across, and there's no 'normal' size. People are sometimes worried by the little 'blobs' which often run round the areola but these are perfectly normal structures called 'the tubercles of Montgomery'.

The nipple itself contains the openings of the 15–20 milk ducts which are directly connected to one of the most important emotional regions of your brain. That's one reason why both suckling a baby *and* sexual stimulation of the nipple both tend to have a very immediate emotional impact on almost all women.

The Male Nipple

A man's nipple is a sexually excitable organ. That's because it comes from the same basic tissues which go to form the *female* nipple, and has much the same nerve supply. The only thing that makes the female nipple different is that female hormones have made it grow and develop – and made the breast form around it.

If you give a man female hormones, he too will develop female-looking nipples and breasts.

The fact that the ordinary male's nipple has such a rich nerve supply means that a woman can produce a very good reaction in her partner by stroking it, kissing it, or teasing it gently with her tongue – in fact, just what most women like men to do to *their* nipples.

Nipple erection

When a woman becomes sexually aroused, the nipple promptly starts to stand out. US sex researchers Johnson and Masters say that it may lengthen by as much as a centimetre. But just before orgasm, the surrounding areola also becomes rather engorged – which is why the nipple appears less prominent at that moment.

Why should the nipple become erect anyway? The only reason I can think of is that it's an undoubted fact that the erect nipple is more sexually attractive.

That's why the female nude is traditionally depicted with erect nipples. Renoir's *blondes baigneuses*, today's pin-ups, and the showgirls of Paris are all part of this tradition, Indeed, in Paris theatres they're supposed to keep a feather in the wings – so that the performers can go on stage in a suitably outstanding condition . . .

Q For some time now, I have been extremely irritated about seeing naked or half-naked females on films, TV and video. My boyfriend doesn't agree with me, but I think that it is unbalanced and unfair to show nude women and not nude men. I feel that if they show one, they ought to show the other – otherwise, it's degrading to women. What is your opinion?

A I'm inclined to agree with you. Quite a lot of women – though certainly not all – do like looking at naked men, and I don't see why their wishes should be frustrated. In fact, I *am* available for ladies' luncheon parties.

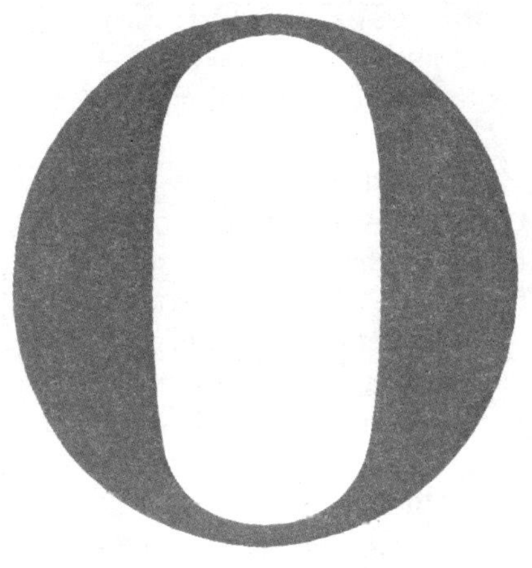

Open Marrriage

Quite a few people these days are perfectly agreeable to their partners sleeping with other folk. Where a couple reach such an arrangement with each other, it's called an 'open marriage'.

It all sounds very civilized and sophisticated, but often it *doesn't* work out: maybe one partner gets jealous or even violent, or perhaps one or other party will fall in love with someone they've bedded. And then there are dangers of infection and 'outside' pregnancy.

Furthermore, if you have children, it can be very unsettling for them to observe – as they're almost certain to do – that some nights Mummy sleeps with Bill, or Fred, or Jim, or Pierre, or Helmut . . .

Rather reluctantly, I have to say that some open (or, at least fairly open) marriages work. An alleged example was that of the late and much-loved Lord Louis Mountbatten and his immensely-admired wife Edwina. But the success of that highly unusual relationship depended on the fact that Mountbatten was almost totally devoid of jealousy, and apparently didn't mind in the least whether his wife actually decided to give herself to their close friend Prime Minister Nehru or not.

From personal observation of people who have tried to work an open marriage policy, I'd say that very few couples could have achieved that kind of non-jealous harmony. I'd even go further and say that most open marriages are likely to end in open divorce.

Q I am a reader in the Middle East. I do not know much about sex. I would like to know if any health problems could be caused by swallowing sperms.

A Well, ma'am, it's not everybody's cup of tea (so to speak), but plenty of women do it. It's certainly not dangerous to your health – but whether it's against the law in the Middle East, I just wouldn't know.

Q I'm in love with a gorgeous male. The problem is that I get so wet and slippery before we start to make love. There is so little friction that sometimes he can't reach a climax.

Is there anything I could do to control the excessive production of 'love juices?'

A 'Fraid not. But he could use a sheath – preferably a 'ribbed' one – which would give more friction.

Another trick is to put your legs together (i.e. between his) during love-making; this 'squeezes' him very slightly and should help to increase the friction.

In fact, if your relationship settles down, you'll probably find that you no longer have quite such violent outpourings of secretion as soon as he gets near you.

Q My husband shouts so loud while climaxing that I'm afraid he can be heard at the end of the road.

He says he shouts because sex is marvellous – and gets better and better! Is this sort of reaction common in men?

A Not really, ma'am. Women do mostly shriek – or at least squeak – when they reach orgasm. But the majority of blokes just gasp or groan a bit.

Still, I think it's great that your husband is so appreciative of your charms – especially as I understand he's in his 60s!

Orgasm

At the medical journal where I work, we still get a steady flow of letters from a small number of doctors who firmly believe that women do not reach an orgasm.

This is manifestly not true! Female orgasm is a widespread and – it would appear – intensely pleasurable event. Judging by the descriptions which women give ('The moment when all the fuses blow', and so on), it seems to be just as nice for you as male orgasm is for us men.

Studies by the amazing sex researchers Virginia Johnson and Dr William Masters – who carried out some truly exotic lab experiments with intra-vaginal cameras and whatnot – seem to confirm without the slightest doubt that most women do reach a climax, in the sense of a dramatic and delightful discharge in the nervous system, in much the same way as men do.

Indeed, the experiments of Johnson and Masters (please note the careful non-sexist reversal of their names!) taught us more about the physiology of female climaxes than we'd ever known before.

Women have a great advantage over men in that – in theory at least – they're capable of second, third, fourth, or fifth climaxes in quick succession. For most men, that's just a pipe dream (if you'll forgive the phrase).

But don't let's get this business of multiple orgasm out of proportion. Kinsey's statistics indicated that only about one woman in seven went in for these multiple climaxes. I'd say that a few more women have multiple orgasms today, but most are perfectly happy with one orgasm at a time, thank you very much.

Now we have to face the fact that there are also many women who *don't* reach a climax, and who are often very upset about it. About 20% of young married women say that they have not yet experienced an orgasm – though the percentage is far smaller among women of more mature years.

I would like to dispose of the old myth that orgasm is supposed to originate from stimulation of one part of your body only – and that anything else is 'wrong'.

Your nervous system can blow its top as a result of stimulation of your vagina, your clitoris, your G-spot, your buttocks, or your breasts – or indeed your ears, if enough sweet nothings are whispered into them. Whatever turns you on, enjoy it!

Multiple Orgasm

People do get either very excited or very upset about this business of multiple orgasm. When **SHE** published an article about *male* multiple orgasm, it aroused great interest – and also some indignation that the subject should be mentioned at all.

Well, what's the truth about *female* multiple orgasm? Does it happen? If so, how many times can it happen? What proportion of women 's experience it? And does it matter if you don't experience it?

Let me answer that last question first. If you don't have multiple orgasms, it doesn't matter two hoots. It doesn't matter how many times you can 'ring the bell' – what counts is whether you're *happy* with your sex life.

From what I've said, you'll gather that there really is no physiological doubt that multiple organsm does happen in some women. The extraordinary laboratory experiments of Johnson and Masters (not to mention their indefatigable – and improbable – vaginal camera) in the USA have made this quite clear.

So how many climaxes can a woman have? Anecdotal evidence indicates that under the right circumstances, three, four or five orgasms would be quite common.

With the help of a skilled lover, it's certainly quite easy for a very small proportion of women to knock up (say) 15 or 20 climaxes in a single night – though they do tend to feel a bit flaked out next day!

I have heard fantastic tales of the occasional very passionate woman being able to have 100 or even 200 orgasms in an evening, though it's very hard to know whether to place any credence in such claims.

Now to the crunch question. What proportion of women do genuinely experience multiple orgasms?

It' not easy to answer that one. Dr Kinsey's researches on American women back in 1953 suggested that only about one woman in seven could have multiple climaxes.

But that was a long time ago, and women have generally become much less inhibited since then. Ms Shere Hite's recent US sex surveys seem to suggest that a rather higher proportion of women had multiple orgasms. And our recent **SHE** surveys indicate that many British women reach multiple orgasm IF they're adequately stimulated.

Female Orgasm

Let me set out the physiological facts, as discovered by the intrepid team of Masters and Johnson.

What happens at orgasm is this. At the supreme moment of pleasure, most of the muscles of your body go into a quite uncontrollable spasm.

During that period of the orgasm when your eyes are open, your pupils can be seen to be big and dreamy – this is an effect of adrenaline, coursing through your bloodstream.

Your face – could you but see it, dear reader – contorts into an expression which may be like the widest of smiles, but which more commonly is almost like a grimace of pain. But of course, it's not pain that causes it – it's ecstasy (I hope).

Even your toes curl up with pleasure – one of the most reliable signs of orgasm to anyone who happens to be in the regions of a woman's feet at the moment of climax (unusual, I'll admit).

What else? The mouth of your vagina – which has become swollen into a sort of soft collar intended to fit snugly round the base of your man's penis – now starts to contract in a series of highly pleasureable waves.

These waves occur roughly once a second – that is, with much the same frequency as the 'surges' of a man's climax. Several readers have misunderstood what I said about these vaginal contractions, and thought I was claiming they didn't happen. Yes – they do occur: but the point is that a man can't normally feel them (which is why it's so easy for a woman to fake orgasm).

Elsewhere in the book, on the pages headed 'clitoral erection' and 'nipple erection', I have explained the breast changes which take place at orgasm. Another orgasmic change is a curious measles-like rash, which briefly appears in fair-skinned women just as they 'come.'

Finally, there's one other event associated with female orgasm – *le cri*. The characteristic 'climax cry' is evinced by most – though not all – women at the very apogee of the climactic experience.

I'm not kidding when I say that this really is a very useful sound – because it does give a man the best possible indication that his loved one has 'got there'.

It's also a curiously disturbing and erotic sound when you hear it through the thin walls of a hotel bedroom. But that's another story.

Male Orgasm

We've already discussed female orgasm. So let's be even-handed and investigate the same function as it occurs in men. How does your man reach *his* orgasm?

Well, the extraordinary lab experiments of Johnson and Masters in the US have shown that there are quite a few similarities between male and female orgasms. For instance, a bloke has his climax in four basic stages, just as a woman does.

The excitement phase is simply the one in which he has achieved an erection and is getting more and more enthusiastic about you.

The plateau phase is the one in which he remains more or less in control of himself, but could 'fire off' at any time. In successful relationships, this agreeable plateau can, if wished, be prolonged for half an hour or more.

The ejaculation phase is of course very brief, and corresponds to what you experience at the height of your own orgasm. A man's muscular contractions at this stage occur with much the same frequency as those experienced by a woman.

The resolution phase is the rather pleasant 'afterglow' time, during which the man's sex organs return to their normal state.

You'll notice that after the ejaculation phase, there's what the sexperts call a refractory period. This means the time during which a man cannot respond again, no matter what you do to him. Only after the refractory period is over can he have another climax.

In younger men, the refractory period can be quite short – sometimes only a matter of minutes. In older men, however, it may last some days. I have to say that because of the refractory period, multiple orgasm is rare in gents, although there are a few recorded cases. Multiple orgasm in men is entirely dependent on age.

Indeed, the solid and dependable researches of Dr Kinsey indicate that the percentage of blokes who can reach multiple orgasm at various ages is as follows:

Under 16	20%
16–20	15%
21–30	9%
31–40	6%
41–50	2.5%
51–60	3.5%

I suppose this goes some way toward explaining why so many women today take younger lovers . . .

Q I have a very good marriage, but though I can reach a climax easily through petting, I can't do it during actual sex. Am I abnormal?

A Nope. Several studies carried out over the last few years indicate that – contrary to what's generally believed – most women *don't* usually reach an orgasm during intercourse – only during love play. Women who regularly 'ring the bell' during actual intercourse are fortunate, but in a minority.

Q This is a most embarrassing question, but I would like to sort it out before I marry my fiancé.

The trouble is this. When we dance together, he keeps having a climax in his trousers! We've never had sex together, partly because we're both shy. What could he do to avoid it?

A Has he ever considered wearing a kilt?

Seriously, lots of young chaps have had the embarrassing experience of 'coming' in their pants while dancing with a pretty girl. The friction of the trousers and the pressure of the girl's body can combine to have explosive effects when a nervous young man is on a short fuse.

In other words, he may well have the very common male condition called 'premature ejaculation', or 'hair-trigger trouble'. You won't find this out for certain until you try and make love to him.

The important thing now is to talk to him about it, treating the subject with sympathy and humour.

Meanwhile, if you agree not to bother with dances for a while, this would take the pressure off him (in more ways than one).

Q I am a 21-year-old girl from Ireland and am very shy. I had a boyfriend, but he wanted to make love to me. When I said I didn't want to, he went away.

Since then I have been very depressed. And when I go out, everyone stares at me.

Recently I have taken to cuddling up and 'making love' with a teddy bear, and this brings me to a climax. Is that harmful?

A Would that be the teddy bear with the big smile on his face by any chance?

Seriously, what you've been doing with 'Big Ted' is quite harmless – and I'm sure no-one with any sense would blame you for seeking solace in this way at such a difficult time.

As you say, you're fairly depressed. The feeling that 'everyone is looking at me' is *very* characteristic of depression.

So I do urge you to go and get some help from your doc now. You also need some 'self-assertiveness' training to help you overcome your shyness.

If there isn't a psychologist in your area who offers this kind of training, write to the *Institute of Behaviour Therapy*, who have self-assertiveness tapes and books, and arrange seminars for shy people. The address is: *38, Queen Anne Street, London W1*.

Q I can climax when my husband pets me, but not when we have intercourse, as a rule. Is there something wrong with me?

A Nope. As I've said several times in this column, one of the great myths about sex is that most women regularly climax during intercourse.

The admirable US statistician Ms Shere Hite has shown in her massive American surveys that this is quite untrue. Most women don't reach an orgasm regularly during actual intercourse, as opposed to love-play.

I once had the very enjoyable experience of having tea at the Ritz with Ms Hite, and she made this point very forcefully, over the cucumber sandwiches. (I was profoundly grateful that she didn't order crumpet.)

Q While I was driving along the M6 to visit my husband in Liverpool, I found that I was stroking myself to pass the time away. There was no danger of me losing control of the car, but I did actually reach a climax. Do you think this was wrong?

A Well, as long as it was only the M6 . . . I do understand that the long stretch before the Sandbach turn-off can be more than trifle tedious. But next time you feel a little bored on the motorway, it may prove a little safer just to turn on the radio (rather than yourself).

Q I am 47 years old, happily married for 23 years, and have never had a climax.

Some years ago, I discovered the vibrator. With the use of it, I have been able to experience feelings that I'd never had before.

My heart races, I perspire and pant, and I have to shout out as my legs and body stiffen.

The feeling that I have is quite fantastic. But though I have been to various doctors and sex therapists. I cannot 'click over' into a climax. Please help.

A Well, ma'am to be quite frank, it sounds to me as though what you're having at the moment *is* an orgasm, by most people's definitions.

I know you feel that there's something *more* which you should be experiencing. But people's climaxes do vary a great deal and to a lot of women, what you describe in your letter would be a climax.

I don't think you should keep 'striving' for more: this is rarely productive where orgasms are concerned. To be honest, I think that you're lucky that you're happily married and that you're experiencing sexual sensations which you yourself describe as 'fantastic'.

Q I am a young lady from Cambridge, and I am made to feel inadequate because my boyfriend says that I do not 'come'.

But I think that I do! However, he says that it is impossible for a woman to reach orgasm without gushing forth fluid at the moment of ecstacy.

A It's your boyfriend who's gushing, dear young lady from Cambridge! He's not a St John's man, is he?

Honestly, he's really got this the wrong way round. It has recently been established that a small proportion of women do seem to produce some sort of fluid at the moment of orgasm. But the vast majority do NOT!

So if you think you're 'coming' at Cambridge, I'm sure you're the one who is right.

Q I am usually on the very brink of a climax when my husband 'comes'. He then falls asleep immediately, leaving me frustrated! Do ALL men make a habit of doing this?

A Many do, dear lady. It's thought that immediately after orgasm, a sedative chemical floods through a man's brain – making him very sleepy, unless he fights against it. And that's why it may be a good 10 minutes or so before a man can lift a finger (if you'll forgive the phrase).

However if you stress to your

husband that you really want him to stay awake and 'finish you off', I'm sure he'll try. The alternative would be to buy a vibrator – you never know, the buzzing might wake him up.

Q In answer to your question about being multi-orgasmic, we can only answer that in this household, we do not know. But we would be very interested to find out.

We are two potentially multi-orgasmic females, and as yet we have not found a skilled lover.

If you would like to send one round, we would be willing to try him out, in the aid of scientific research – and we will forward the results of the experiment on to you.

A Would male readers kindly note that I am *not* going to reveal the address of these two scientifically-minded females to anyone! However, I'm grateful to them for demonstrating that British women do have a sense of humour about sex (even in Leicester).

Q I do not reach multiple orgasms. Perhaps you could discuss the subject of oral sex, which more and more men seem to expect. Common sense tells me that all forms of it must be unhygienic.

A Common sense doesn't say anything of the kind, ma'am. It is certainly foolish to go in for oral sex when you have a mouth infection – or indeed, a sex infection.

It is particularly important not to do it when you have a 'cold sore' on the lip, as the virus which causes this is very nearly identical with the one which causes genital herpes.

But vast numbers of women do find oral love-play helpful in giving them orgasms (whether single or multiple), and enriching their sex lives generally. I can't see anything wrong with that.

Q I noticed your recent comment (in the SHE sex survey) about some women reaching orgasm when having their nipples touched.

Surely this is impossible?

I have never attempted to stimulate my wife in this way, because I have always assumed that her breasts (being small) are unresponsive.

A Small breasts are just as sexually responsive as big ones, sir

– so why not give it a go? I'm sure your wife would be pleasantly surprised – after all these years of not having her boobs touched!

I must stress that only a *tiny minority* of women can reach a climax in this way.

But an American survey of 'easily orgasmic women' revealed that 20% of these highly climactic females could 'come' just though having their nipples stroked or licked.

Q How on earth can you fake an orgasm! Surely a man must feel whether the vagina contracts or not at the moment of climax?

A First, I'm afraid that quite a few women do 'fake orgasm'. Regrettably, some doctors still advise them do to it – which I think is crazy.

In fact, it's quite easy to fake a climax. You see you're mistaken in thinking that at the moment of orgasm, the vagina contracts and so gives a signal to the man that climax has occurred. (Several other readers who're written to me have the same erroneous idea.)

Actually, it's extremely difficulty for a man to know with certainty whether a woman has reached a climax. Most men rely on a sort of hopeful guesswork – based on whether their partner's shrieks/groans/moans/whatever appear to be on a *crescendo* or not.

Alas, much of the sexual misunderstanding between male and female is due to the simple fact that many men simply haven't a clue as to whether their partners have 'done it'! Sometimes it's very difficult for gentlemen to follow the ancient rule 'Ladies come first . . . '

Q Re orgasm: I thought some of your readers might take comfort from my story. I am now 25, and for seven years I experienced frustration and depression because I could not 'come'.

At first I faked –though that's difficult when you don't known what you're supposed to be faking – but eventually I resigned myself to the non-event.

However, early last year, the big event *did* happen and afterwards all I could do was cry!

I now enjoy orgasm regularly, and my sex life with my husband is getting better and better. So my message to women is: don't give up.

A That's my message too. Thank you for a delightfully cheery letter. I think it's very important for people to realise that the chances of reaching orgasm increase steadily as a woman gets older. Indeed, the graph is still climbing upwards at age 45, so no woman should ever lose hope.

Q My husband and I don't reach a simultaneous climax. Is this abnormal?

A Stone the crows, ma'am! The Delvin Report showed conclusively that only a minority of **SHE** readers usually 'come' at the same moment as their partners. Contrary to what so many 'bodice-ripper' novels would have us believe, simultaneous orgasm is really not all that common. So you're normal.

Q My fiancée does not reach orgasm during actual intercourse because she says my penis is too small. This is very distressing for me.

A I'm sure it is – and it's very unfortunate that she used this phraseology.

In fact, it's *very* unlikely that your penile size is anything to do with it. As I keep endlessly saying, most women do NOT regularly reach a climax during intercourse itself. So I think the two of you should go to a Family Planning Clinic and ask for: (a) some advice about love play; (b) a 'second opinion' on your phallic dimensions.

Q My problem is that I don't know if I've ever had an orgasm.

A If you don't know – then you haven't. Sorry to be so blunt! But from the rest of your letter, you're obviously very young and not very experienced sexually.

As I've often indicated, it's quite common not to have an orgasm until you've been established for some time in a relationship with a skilled and loving partner. Your day will come. (And so will you.)

Q This is not really a problem, more of a request for information. Should you not believe what I say, then I do not blame you. Some years ago I found out by accident that I could give a woman an orgasm just by holding her hand and using my mind. Later, I progressed to doing it just by holding the tip of a woman's finger and concentrating. And I even found that just by looking

into a woman's eyes. I could make her have an orgasm. Is this a common occurrence, or not?

A No, it's not common – even in Bournemouth, where you're writing from!

Frankly, sir, I'm a little doubtful whether you're serious. But if you really do think you can make women have climaxes just by gazing into their eyes, then I think you should ask yourself whether they're convulsing with orgasms – or with laughter.

Q I can't reach a climax, simply because my stupid husband refuses to accept that he has to stroke my clitoris in order to make me come!

He says that rubbing a woman's clitoris is 'unmanly' and maintains that women ought to be able to climax through intercourse, without any use of the hands.

What can I do?

A Alas ma'am, many men have this delusion – which is why we've included a question on this very subject in our national survey of blokes.

But chaps who are well-read on the subject of the clitoris (I s'pose you could call them the *cliterati*, really) are aware that most women do need skilled manual stimulation of this organ if they are to reach orgasm easily.

Try showing this answer to your thick-witted, obstinate husband. If he *still* won't oblige, then I'm afraid you may have to resort to masturbation or a vibrator.

Q You were wrong when you said that the best indicator that a woman has reached orgasm is her loud cry.

You clearly don't know what you're talking about!

My vagina throbs such a lot that I'm sure any man could feel it and know that I've reached a climax.

A Well, I'm sorry to say that you're mistaken.

It's surprisingly difficult for a man to tell whether his lady has 'come' – unless she cries out.

That's why so many women are successful in faking orgasm – and also why so many blokes keep saying to their lovers: 'Er . . . have you come yet, dear?'

You're quite right in saying that at orgasm, the vagina contracts (about 8 or 10 times – at roughly 0.8 second intervals).

But contrary to what you might think, these 'throbs' aren't easy for a chap to feel – especially as a very sexually-knowledgeable woman may have been deliberately contracting her pelvic muscles powerfully during intercourse.

Laboratory experiments in America (where else?) do show that the changes which take place in a woman's body at the moment of orgasm are either a) not easy to detect; or b) very readily faked.

The main 'orgasm indicators' which have been discovered in these experiments are:

Breasts: soon after orgasm, the previously 'collapsed' nipples start standing out more.
Skin: in many fair-skinned women, a 'sex flush' appear shortly before orgasm – and disappears at the time of climax.
Fingers and toes: these often curl up at the moment of orgasm.
Bottom: the muscles of your rear end contract involuntarily two to five times – if the orgasm is very intense.
Womb: this contracts powerfully during orgasm, but it's too high to be detected by the man.

These orgasmic changes were first described by the US sexologists, Virginia Johnson and William Masters – who together observed about 5,000 climaxes during research in the lab. (After which they did the decent thing and got married!)

Q **When I 'come' with my boyfriend, I wet myself. He is very understanding, saying it's natural and he doesn't mind. But I do!**

A I don't believe there's anything you can do about it – so I think it'd be better for you to try and adopt his sensible attitude.

Very large numbers of women do produce a fluid at the moment of orgasm. There's a lot of controversy about the nature of this fluid – which may be urine, or a secretion produced by the famous female 'G-spot'.

What is not controversial is that it is natural for these women to 'ejaculate' at orgasm.

Also, do bear in mind that some men find this phenomenon a very considerable 'turn on' – and a useful indicator that the lady really has come (see below).

Q **Men never seem to know whether I have reached orgasm or not. What is the best 'indicator' to tell them to look out for?**

A The cry ! There are various other physiological signs of

reaching a climax, but you'd need to be a very sharp-eyed sexologist to notice them.

So if you want to tell your man that you've got there, shriek loudly! (It'd also be a help if you seized the first available moment to say 'I've come . . .')

Q I was astounded to discover that most women don't reach a climax during intercourse.

I always do, and my husband and I *often* climax simultaneously. We have been married for 16 years, and I can count on one hand the number of times I haven't climaxed.

I thought that what we experienced was common to most couples. So it was only after reading your column that I realised how incredibly lucky we are.

A Too right. Until very recently, everybody from psychiatrists to readers of romantic fiction seemed to assume that most women automatically reached orgasm during intercourse itself – usually at the same time as their blokes did.

But the famous American sex researcher Ms Shere Hite (author of *The Hite Report*) rocked everybody by discovering that only about 30% of US women regularly reached orgasm during actual intercourse.

Since then, several large British surveys run by newspapers and magazines have shown that the figure for this country is about 30% to 40%.

However, I'd like to make clear that this *doesn't* mean that the rest of the female population aren't having an orgasm at all. It's just that they're mainly reaching it through love play.

Q I'm a mother of five children, and I'm extremely embarrassed by the fact that when I climax with my husband, I pass wind! Any ideas?

A Quite a common complaint – mainly due to the way the pelvic muscles tend to become slack after childbirth.

You may not be able to defeat your orgasm-flatulent problem completely. But 'pelvic' floor exercises might well help you to achieve better control over your wayward bottom?

Fortunately, the pelvic exercises which **SHE** popularised in conjuction with the self-help group SHAPE are now being taught in gyms and fitness studios.

I suggest you go along to the

nearest one and get yourself a pelvic toning-up course.

Q Can it really be true that some women are able to reach orgasm just through having their nipples rubbed! My husband says he once knew a girl who could do this, but I don't believe him.

A Well, ma'am, I *do* believe him – because it can happen.

But the ability to reach a climax through breast stimulation alone is unusual. So there's no need for you to feel inadequate because you can't peform the same difficult feat.

Q Whenever my partner and I make love, I find that the pressure tickles my bladder. So, if love-making carries on too long, I have to stop to go to the loo. I'd be grateful for any suggestions.

A Common problem, ma'am, I'm afraid. I think that all you can do is try to switch to other positions, in which the male organ doesn't press on the bladder or the urinary pipe.

One such posture is the 'lateral' in which your guy lies on his left side next to you, while you lie on your back with thighs raised – often known as 'having a bit on the side'.

Another useful trick would be to make sure that you remember to spend a penny before you start to make love, so that your bladder is completely empty.

Q Until just lately, I had a girl-friend in our town who claimed to reach 25 orgasms in a night – and she certainly *seemed* to when I was in bed with her. This was all a bit much for me, and we recently split up. But I wonder – was she faking?

A I doubt it. Though most women are happy with just one climax, there are quite a few who can knock off 20 or 25 in a session. You, sir, did very well to help her achieve such figures – and you've nothing to be ashamed of if she got a bit much for you to handle. (Note to male readers: no, gentlemen, I am not revealing any clues as to where this talented female resides.)

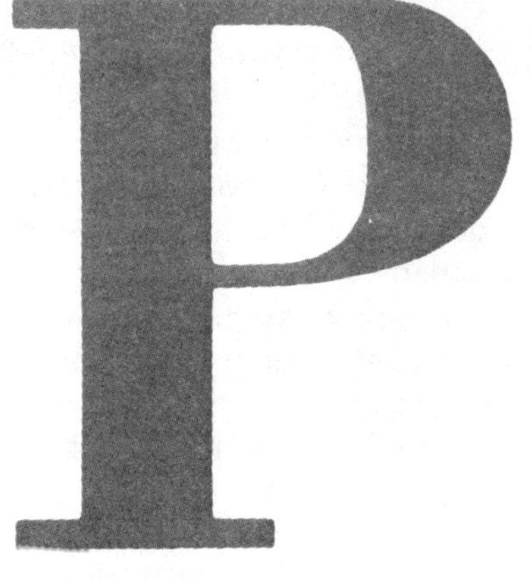

Q **I have always regarded myself as a very feminine and fastidious woman, so I am distressed by something I can't seem to control. It is very embarrassing, and it's this – I can't help passing wind in bed, specially when making love. What can I do?**

A Well, I'm not going to joke about this, because it can be a very upsetting problem. I've had a number of letters from women who are troubled by 'the wind', especially during pregnancy.

The only anti-gas measures I know of are the following:

cut right down on any fibre-containing food, including peas, beans and almost anything advocated by the F-Plan (!) Diet

try nibbling charcoal biscuits – these are obtainable without prescription from many chemists

if possible, sit on the loo for a good ten minutes before you go to bed – particularly if love-making is contemplated

But honestly, I think the most important thing is to talk this over with your man. If you can both laugh about it – rather than taking it seriously – then it will cease to matter.

Pelvic Floor

What put me in mind of this structure was a conversation I had with an intelligent and well-informed woman who thought that pelvic floor exercises were so-called because you had to do them on the floor.

The pelvic floor is a sort of cleverly-interwoven basket of muscle which forms a network that supports all the organs in your pelvis – including your womb, your ovaries and your bladder.

You can get a rough idea of the size and shape of the muscles of the pelvic floor by simply holding your two hands palms upwards in front of you. Then slide the two hands together, so that the fingers interlock. The resulting shallow 'basin' is quite like the pelvic floor. Imagine that it's supporting your pelvic organs – and imagine too that (as in the anatomical drawing) there are two apertures in the 'basin', through which pass the vagina and the rectum.

Now it's important that all women should know about this pelvic floor musculature. Why? Because in so many, many females, childbirth leads to serious *weakening* of these muscles – with unfortunate consequences for your love-life and your health.

Repeated childbirth and *prolonged or difficult* labours are particularly likely to do this to a mother.

As far as her sex life is concerned, she's likely to find that her vagina seems to have become slack and loose. Either she or her bloke (or both) are liable to feel dissatisfied because things aren't as 'snug' as they once were.

The second consequence of pelvic floor slackness may be on the woman's health. After some years, severe weakness of these muscles can lead to prolapse (descent of the womb); much more frequently it simply causes problems with urination the woman finds that she has embarrassing incontinence, especially when she coughs or laughs.

Happily, gross weakness of the pelvic floor muscles can usually be put right with one of a variety of surgical 'repair operations'. But obviously, it's much better to avoid surgery altogether, and this can be done by means of pelvic floor exercises.

Every woman should do these exercises daily for several months after the birth of a child, in order to prevent prolapse and the other troubles I've mentioned. Even when you've *already* got a good deal of pelvic floor weakness, its amazing how six months of Kegel exercises alone can often put things right. Ideally, every newly-delivered mother ought to be taught the exercises I'm going to describe. And any woman who feels that her vagina is a little too loose can do them too; they're quite good fun and they may prevent you from needing a vaginal 'repair' operation later on in life.

The exercises are called 'Kegel exercises', after the bloke who invented them.

The two exercises can and should be done during intercourse: this is enjoyable, for both of you. Why? Because once you've got these 'love muscles' developed a bit, you'll discover that doing the exercises creates an agreeable sort of 'milking' sensation in his male organ. (You don't get this kind of advice in other books, you know!)

But its no good just doing the two exercises during lovemaking. As with any other 'muscle building' exercises, you need to do them for about 20 minutes, twice a day – over at least six months. But here's the good news: you can do the exercises while you're at work, while you're pushing a pram, while you're sitting in the bath, while you're talking to the vicar, or whatever – no-one will know.

Exercise one: make a real effort to contract the *front* part of your pelvic muscles, by 'tightening up' as if you were trying to stop yourself passing water. Hold the contraction for ten seconds, then release for ten seconds, for ten minutes.

Exercise two: make a similar effort to contract the *back* part of your pelvic floor muscles by 'tightening up' as if to hold back a bowel movement. Again, maintain the contraction for ten seconds, then relax for ten. Repeat for ten minutes.

There are now at least four devices which are supposed to help people do Kegel exercises. The Gynatone is an acrylic vaginal cylinder to which you can attach successively greater weights as your vaginal muscles become stronger (seriously!). The Femtone is a simple isometric vaginal exerciser. Its makers also produce two much more complicated biofeedback-type devices; one of them converts your vaginal muscle contractions into electrical impulses and records them on a chart – and the other (incredibly enough) plays them back to you on a loudspeaker.

The Penis

The penis the organ which is the subject of an amazing amount of emotion and embarrassment and even outrage. Strange really, because it's a somewhat unimpressive little structure, comparing rather unfavourably in dimemsions with a decent-sized *andouillette*.

However, one has to face the fact that many men and women do have hang-ups about the penis. In the case of men, vast numbers of them have an extraordinary obsession about penile *size*.

In the case of women , a surprising number of females feel frightened or disgusted by the idea of a close encounter with a male organ. Some wives are so emotional about this matter that they cannot touch their husband's penises.

So it seems to me that life would be a great deal easier if everybody understood a few of the basic facts about this organ and how it works. Here goes!

The penis is the male equivalent of a woman's clitoris. So it's equipped with a great many pleasure receptors which, when stimulated, produce very agreeable sensations in the brain.

Now the average penis in its non-erect state is quite a bit smaller than most people imagine. Your average bloke measures between just over three inches (8.5 cm) and just over four (10.5 cm) when he's in this state – but it varies a lot, depending on the weather.

And the US sex researchers Masters and Johnson have discovered a curious fact of which few men are aware. Though penises vary quite a bit in size in the non-erect state, they're nearly all about the same size when they're erect – six and a half inches. So though many males feel inadequate about the size of their phalluses, this is all quite unnecessary – especially as most women aren't remotely interested in the size of a man's organ anyway.

The penis is a very simple structure in comparison with the female genital organ. Really it just consists of three cylinders of tissue, which are capable of filling with blood (thus causing an erection) when a man thinks about sex.

On the end of these three cylinders is the cone-shaped glans, which is the most sexually sensitive part. Hence the phrase: 'The Devil makes work for idle glans . . . ' Really, the only other thing to say about the penis is that contrary to what so many women (and men) imagine, it is actually a pretty *clean* structure. Provided a man washes regularly under his foreskin (if present) there should be nothing 'dirty' about his penis at all.

Amputation of the Penis

First, some good news. A treatment is now available for one of the most tragic accidents which can befall a boy or a man.

Because it's a somewhat vulnerable part of the body, the male organ can all too easily be chopped off in an accident. Also a few boys are born without the organ, and some men lose it through cancer or burns.

But at the East Virginia Medical School in America, plastic surgeons have developed a technique for fashioning a penis out of skin flaps taken from other parts of the body.

The method enables the patient to feel at least some sensation from his new penis. In one case, the establishment of sensation in the new organ has been so good that the young man in question has been able to achieve intercourse and even orgasm.

At the time of writing, I'm not aware that the operation has been attempted in Britain.

Q Is it really true that sex feels different if you do it with someone of another race?

A Not as far as I am aware. There are many myths about this – some of which, alas, are part of the obscene folklore of racial prejudice.

From a purely medical point of view, I'd say that I've noticed no structural differences between the sex organs of all the various races, so there's no particular reason why it should feel different.

Q We are three hairdressers in Exmouth, and we (and our customers) are a bit bewildered by the connection between a man's sexual performance the size of his penis.

So what we want to know is this: what is normal size? Please enlighten us, or we'll be forced to get out our rulers.

A I don't think that's a good idea! But many readers have written in saying they don't know what average size is. So here are the full, unexpurgated figures.

The average chap usually measures about three and a half

inches (that's 9 cm) in the resting condition – but much less in January because it's so chilly (even down in Exmouth).

When erect, the average bloke's measurement is six and half inches ($16\frac{1}{2}$ cm).

In fact, sexologists have been able to discover that 'resting' measurements are pretty irrelevant – because most penises tend to be very roughly the same size when they're erect, give or take an inch or two.

Now I would like to make one very serious point.

Most women are not aware of the fact that the average chap goes through life feeling a bit sexually inadequate because he's convinced his organ is on the small side. Even gentlemen equipped with eight inches (20.5 cm) or more can have this delusion!

Indeed, I actually get letters from guys terrified to take off their clothes in front of a woman – in case she laughs. There are chaps whose sex lives have been blighted permanently because somebody once thoughtlessly said to them: 'Your willy's not very big, is it?'

So dear readers, do try and avoid making that kind of morale-crumbling remark! We are, after all, an insecure and vulnerable sex . . .

Q I am a girl of 18, and I just keep feeling very dirty and guilty because of the fact that when I was about 11 or 12, I let my brother play around with me. Does this make me perverted?

A Not at all. There's a vast amount of this sort of childish experimentation around, so you're not abnormal in any way.

The best thing would be to forget all about it. But if it keeps preying on your mind, go and have a chat with your local *Brook Advisory Centre for Young People*.

Perversion

Different people mean entirely different things by this word. It's been shown that where a person hasn't had very much education, he's more likely to regard perfectly normal sexual activity as being 'wrong'. Even today, there are quite a few people around who think that any love-making between husband and wife other than intercourse in the 'standard' position is 'perverted'.

However, most people are rather better-informed than this, and the necessity for various types of love-play between husband and wife is generally recognized. Doctors in the field of sexual medicine do not regard any mutually-satisfying activity which is not harmful as being 'perverted'.

Psychological Illnesses

There are, however, true perversions, some of which are physically dangerous – sadism, masochism, and so on. A characteristic feature of all these is that the patient only wants satisfaction through his or her deviation and not through intercourse. Quite obviously, these are psychological illnesses which should be treated by a psychiatrist, if the patient will agree. (If he *won't* agree and you think he's dangerous, then ditch him –fast!)

Pheromone Production

'Wot on earth are pheromones?' I hear you cry.

Well, they're sex scents, actually. And they're pronounced '*fear*—oh-mones'.

They're delicate aromas which we all produce – so delicate in fact, that other people are scarcely (if at all) conscious of receiving them.

Yet their influence on other folk's sexual behaviour is said to be profound. For instance, the woman who produces a lot of female pheromones is believed to exert an unusually strong attraction on men.

And vice versa: the bloke who produces a lot of male pheromones may have what seems to be an inexplicable charm for women.

It's an interesting theory. And it may explain why in any gathering, there are certain people who are not especially beautiful or handsome in a physical way – yet who seem to be irresistible to the opposite sex.

Pheromones certainly play a very important sexual role in the rest of the animal kingdom. A lot of creatures are drawn to their potential mates by these scents.

Indeed, the most extreme example of pheromone attraction occurs in the pre-mating behaviour of the Emperor moth (*Eudia pavonia*). According to the estimable annual reference work published by Messrs Guinness, the female puts out a pheromone which can be detected by the amorous male at the almost unbelievable distance of 6.8 miles! Human pheromones do not travel such vast distances, but are said to be able to exert their attraction across the proverbial crowded room.

It's not entirely clear which parts of the body produce them, but most are said to be generated by tiny glands in the genital, mouth and armpit areas.

In recent years, shrewd manufactures have 'bottled' male and female pheromones – extracted from animals – in aerosol sprays. These are now quite widely advertised in classified columns and amazing claims are made for their alleged attractant powers. The makers claim that if you spray male pheromones on certain chairs in a room, all the woman who come in will choose those chairs.

Unfortunately, the only demonstration I've ever seen of this alleged effect ended in a complete shambles – mainly because the demonstrator was so plastered that he couldn't remember which chairs he'd sprayed with what.

However, whether the commercially produced pheromone aerosols really do work or not, there seems to be reasonable evidence that the woman who produces a lot of female pheromone is unusually attractive to men.

Q My sex life with my fiancé is fantastic, but I only climax when I'm making love astride him. This worries me.

A You're very lucky to be able to reach a climax during intercourse at all. Be glad of this! When you're married a few years, you'll probably find that climaxes will result from other positions too.

Q I'm about to have a hip replacement. My husband and I used to like to complete our lovemaking with me sitting on him, but at present I can't because of pain. Will it be possible again once I've had the op?

A Almost certainly, ma'am, if the op goes well (as it usually does). P'raps you'd like to write and tell me if you've been able to get back to your old position again?

You might like to know that the French call your favourite posture *'La Diligence de Narbonne'* ('The Narbonne Stagecoach') – because of the powerful bumping sensation it produces.

Q I get tremendous pleasure from being made love to 'doggie-fashion' by my husband. Am I abnormal? Is it perhaps that it's because I was born in the Year of the Dog?

A Is it perhaps that you're sending me up, ma'am? Anyway, there's nothing wrong with making love in this way if you want to.

Admittedly, it's not the most romantic of positions (and in my personal view, it's not exactly the most dignified either). But a lot of people find it satisfying. And some women find it more comfortable than the more 'usual' positions.

Q For various reasons, I cannot tolerate my husband making love to me while lying on top of me, face-to-face. My doctor has suggested that a rear entry position would solve the problem, but somehow I feel that this is too 'animal' for me. Have you any suggestions?

A Indeed yes. Many couples find that the face-to-face missionary position doesn't suit – for instance, because the woman is advanced in pregnancy, or because the husband is much heavier than her, or (quite frequently) because the woman feels threatened or unable to control things in this traditional face-to-face posture.

Similarly, many women are unhappy about 'rear entry' positions – which are a little too reminiscent of your friendly neighbourhood spaniel and his hobby for some people's tastes.

The solution lies in the fact that there are literally countless other positions (which surprisingly few couples know about, but which are detailed in text-books on the subject). For example, an excellent and comfortable compromise can be found in the celebrated 'left lateral position' – in which the woman lies on her back with her knees bent, while her man lies on his side alongside her, entering from behind her thighs. This is sometimes jokily known as 'having a bit on the side'.

'Tomorrow,' as Milton so sagaciously remarked in *Lycidas*, 'to fresh woods and postures new'.

Positions

How Many Positions Are There?

One of the nice things about making love is the fact that there are lots and lots of different ways of doing it. You can make love in a wide variety of ways, and so give each other all sorts of differing pleasant sensations.

How many different ways are there? People are forever arguing about this; one person will say with absolute assurance that there are 71 – while another will announce that the ancient Persians discovered no less than 423.

What's the truth? The fact is that there's no *exact* number of positions. It would be possible to make up a list of hundreds and hundreds provided that you were willing to accept that there were only very minor differences between some of them.

It's also important to remember that some of the wilder antics described in certain books are either dangerous or quite impossible for anyone but a pair of Olympic gymnasts. To take an extreme instance, the oft-quoted example of making love 'swinging from a chandelier' is clearly utter nonsense. (One wonders how many aristocractic families have ruined their best light fixtures this way . . .)

On a more practical level, some of the 'man leaning back' positions mentioned in certain ancient texts are very likely to strain a man's spine – and possibly fracture his penis too! I jest not. Leaning back too far while making love can have disastrous consequences. But rest assured that all the positions mentioned in this chapter are quite safe.

Why Bother with All These Different Positions Anyway?

That's a good question. And the fact is that if you're happy making love in just one single position, and both of you are perfectly satisfied, then that's fine! Carry on doing it the same way.

But the fact is that most people do like a reasonable amount of variety in their love-making. They find that trying out various positions prevents dullness creeping in. (And dullness is something that can cause a lot of problems in marriage.)

They also find that trying out something different gives them all sorts of pleasant new sensations. Sometimes these sensations can help a woman to respond far better than she did before. Sometimes too, they will even help her reach a climax – when previously she had difficulty in doing so.

Furthermore, some women find that sex in an 'ordinary' position is uncomfortable or even painful. (This is particularly common when the male partner is much heavier than the wife.) In these circumstances, a change to an alternative position may well solve the problem.

Incidentally, women who have a 'retroverted' womb – that is, one that points backwards – sometimes find that they have to try out all sorts of love-making positions before they discover one that's really comfortable.

But the main reason why people do like to try out different positions is that it just happens to be fun . . .

Love-making Positions and Fertility

Does the position in which you make love affect your chances of getting pregnant? There are two points to bear in mind here.

Firstly, a lot of people still have the idea that if you make love in a standing position, then pregnancy is impossible. This is nonsense – you can start a baby in any position.

But the second point is very important for couples who have difficulty in conceiving. If your fertility is as bit below par and you're trying for a baby, you should take care to choose love-making positions which give the man's sperm the best possible chance of entering the womb.

For instance, a woman whose womb is retroverted stands the best chance of getting pregnant if she makes love in one of the 'face down' positions described later in this chapter.

This is because a 'face down' position will make the neck of her womb dip into the pool of sperm which forms at the top of her vagina after her partner has reached his climax.

Many infertility clinics advise women with retroverted wombs to have intercourse on all fours, with the man behind them – and to stay in this admittedly somewhat undignified posture for about 10 minutes afterwards.

In contrast, women whose wombs point in the normal direction are usually advised by infertility clinics to have sexual intercourse in one of the 'face up' positions – preferably with a couple of pillows under her bottom, so as to encourage the sperm to stay at the top of the vagina, in contact with the neck of the womb.

Love-making Positions, Arthritis and Disability

From my problem page postbag. I have learned over the years that knowledge of a variety of love-making positions can be a surprising help to people with arthritis, as well as to people with certain other disabilities.

For instance, it's very common for a woman who has arthritis of the hips, but who is otherwise still fit and sexy, to find that the pain and stiffness in her hips make it impossible for her to lie back and make love in the traditional or 'missionary' positon.

A lot of women who have this problem have written to me asking if there's any other position which wouldn't give them pain. Very frequently, a simple change to, say, the 'Spoons' position is enough to solve the problem.

Similarly, men and women who are disabled by back problems, or even by paralysis of a limb, often find that they can still make love with their partners by choosing a position in which their disability is no longer a handicap.

To take one light-hearted example, I can remember a woman who had broken both her legs, and who therefore had to spend several months with her two lower limbs immobile in plaster. She was, however, very keen on making love with her husband – and she managed to continue to do it regularly by going in for an energetic version of the 'cross-buttock' position position described later in this section.

Love-making Positions and Pregnancy

The one time when vast numbers of women really do need to try out other positions is during pregnancy.

From about the middle of pregnancy onwards, it becomes increasingly difficult for a woman to bear the weight of a man on her tummy. These days, many couples make love far into the eighth or even ninth month of pregnancy. And at *that* stage, sex in the missionary position is getting perilously near to impossible.

Mothers-to-be are therefore well advised to try out some of the positions to which I have indicated as being good in pregnancy in this section – particularly those in which the man enters from the side or from behind.

The Positions Most Likely to Give Happiness

In a moment we'll embark on the list of positions which I've chosen for this book. They are, in my view, the positions which are most likely to give a loving couple a good deal of pleasure and happiness.

But if you're repelled or appalled by a particular posture (for instance, some people have a deep aversion to all 'rear entry' positions because of their canine associations), then you shouldn't bother with it: move on to something else instead.

What you'll *not* find in this section are daft, dangerous or impossible positions – though I must admit that it's a bit of a temptation to include one or two of the more bizarre ones I have encountered in my researches.

Face to Face, with Man Above

The first and most common position of love-making is of course the so-called 'missionary' position – the one in which the woman lies flat on her back with her knees raised, while the man lies between her thighs.

This is a pleasant and comfortable position which suits most people very well. Most important is the obvious fact that the couple can kiss each other on the lips while making love. They can also talk to each other – something which isn't terribly easy with the more exotic postures!

Sex books always allege that the history of the position's name is that the white missionaries of Victorian days recommended it to their native converts. I've no idea whether this is true – but if so, I think it says a great deal for the good sense of the missionaries! For this is a very nice, warm, snuggly position, with what sexologists like to call 'a good degree of penetration'.

There are, however, a couple of drawbacks to the missionary position. One is that it's a little difficult for the man to reach the woman's clitoris with his fingertips. (So if it's important to you to have your clitoris stimulated during love-making, you might like to try some of the 'rear entry' positions described later in this section.

The other drawback is that if the man is much heavier than the woman, the missionary posture can be quite uncomfortable, or even painful, for her. The same may be true if she's pregnant. In these circumstances, a sideways or rear entry position my be both more comfortable and more fun.

Finally, I ought to mention that a surprising number of men do have a bit of trouble with the missionary position because they lose their erections just as they try to get 'on top'.

A woman should bear in mind that a man who's a little uncertain about his erection may perform better if he's flat on his back.

Variations on the Missionary Position

A very good idea is to put a couple of pillows under your bottom, so as to tilt it upwards. This decidedly alters the sensations which you and your partner will experience in the missionary position, mainly because you'll find that penetration is deeper. Putting a hot-water bottle under the woman's buttocks has a similar effect.

The next position is *Toulouse*. It's very similar to the missionary position – except that the man's legs are *outside* the woman's. This may seem a rather trivial point, but in fact, the sensations produced by this position are rather different. And – very important – the position is quite useful for the many women who find that child-bearing has made their vaginas lax. This is because the fact that the woman's thighs are *inside* the man's enables her to use her thigh muscles to hold him more snugly – which is nicer for both of them, as a rule.

A thid position in this group is *Béziers*. It's really very like the missionary position – except that the woman spreads her legs out as widely as possible. A lot of ladies find a great deal of sensuous pleasure from this cat-like, 'stretching' position.

Women who own four-poster beds may actually curl their feet around the bedposts. And couples who have a liking for mild forms of bondage may actually go in for tying the woman's ankles to the bedposts. (*Warning:* bondage is most certainly *not* everybody's cup of tea.)

The next 'face to face with male above' position is *Bagnères*. This is a natural development of the missionary position – except that the lady missionary brings her legs up and wraps them round the man's waist.

The lady has to be fairly fit and supple to be able to do this, but the resulting position is good fun for both partners. The altered tilt of the woman's pelvis will usually produce interesting new sensations for both of them.

And so on to *Avignon* where once again, the woman has her legs wrapped round her man's waist – but here he has to *kneel* on the bed (or whatever). If the man is a trifle too enthusiastic there's a slight tendency for his repeated thrusts to keep banging the lady's skull against the headboard of the bed; however, this can be guarded against by skilful placing of the pillows.

The *Narbonne* position is similar but, the man now kneels on the floor behind her, while she (also kneeling) rests her top on the edge of the bed or whatever.

Once again, the over-enthusiastic lover must take care not to be too violent – or he may propel both bed and partner straight across the room and into the nearest wall.

The *Bordeaux* position is an interesting one, but only suitable for the woman with a really supple spine. Lying on her back on the bed, the lady draws her legs up really far, so that she's able to put them over the man's shoulders.

This somewhat exotic position will almost certainly give her all sorts of unusual and even bizarre sensations. The man will probably quite enjoy it too. He should take things very gently, because penetration is very deep indeed in this position.

This position is probably best avoided in late pregnancy, because of the depth of penetration achieved. And I certainly wouldn't recommend it for the sexually inexperienced woman, who might quite reasonably take fright at being asked to assume such an acrobatic pose.

Last in this 'Face to face, male superior' group is the *Montois*, in which the man lies with his body across the woman's, and at 90° to it. In this position, the woman may achieve various interesting sensations, because the man's penis is pressing against the *side* of her vagina. In a variation on this position, the man only turns his body through 45 instead of 90 degrees. This is somewhat improbably known as the 'half cross-buttock'.

Face to Face, with Woman Above

Now we come to the first group of 'female superior' positions. There are still a few men who think that these positions are somehow demeaning to the dignity of the male sex – but I'm sure that their opinions may be safely discounted.

Let's begin with the simple *La Voulte* position. The woman lies on top of the man – in this case with her legs outside his.

This is really a most comfortable position, particularly if the woman is much lighter than her partner. Men appreciate it too – especially as there's a sort of suggestion that the female is seducing the male by making love to him in this way.

To get into this position, all you really need do is this. First, make sure your partner has an erection (sounds silly, but you'd be surprised at how often this elementary preliminary is neglected), then gently throw a leg across his thighs, and climb on top – if necessary, using your hand to guide him in.

In an obvious variation of this position, the woman has her legs *inside* the man's. This is *Carcassonne*. As with the equivalent 'male superior' position this position gives a snug fit – which may be helpful to the couple if the woman's pelvic muscles are a little loose because of childbearing.

Another useful 'female superior' position is *Brive*. It's also called the 'frog' – and I *think* I christened this myself in an earlier book of mine (though if somebody else thought of the name first, I apologize). I hasten to add that the expression 'frog position' has no Gallic overtones, and isn't meant to imply that this particular posture is favoured in the land of the can-can. It just means that you both spread your legs in a breast stroke-type way, so that your pubic regions are pushed together. This is another of those positions which isn't specially romantic, but does often give extremely good sexual sensations.

Another extremely useful female superior position is *Perpignan*. Its quite easy for a woman to get into this position by simply kneeling down *astride* her man, (who is lying flat on his back).

Now this position is very nice but why do I call it 'useful'? Simply because couples who have minor or even major sex difficulties are often advised to try it. The main reason for this is that the position puts no pressure on the woman: if (as is very common) she's a little frightened of intercourse, or tends to panic when the tip of a penis enters her body, then this position leaves her *in control*. She can withdraw a little whenever she wants to – and in effect take charge of the whole act of love if that's what she feels happiest with.

It's easy to develop other positions from this one: for instance, the woman can put one or indeed both legs out to the side (depending how supple she is), and so vary the sensations she feels.

Women who are good at yoga can cross their legs in front of them – across the man's chest. It's even possible to adopt the famed 'lotus position' – though it might be as well to support yourself with your hands while you do this, for fear of falling over and perhaps giving your man a badly sprained penis!

The *Lyon* position is really just one stage on from *Perpignan*. The woman stretches her legs out in front of her, so that she's really sitting on him (facing him) as he lies on his back. She can really move about in the most amazing way in this position, giving both herself and the man a lot of pleasure.

Clearly, the woman can move herself from this position into several closely related ones – for instance, by turning her legs first through 45 degrees and then through 90 degrees in either direction. She can also turn to face away from the man, and then (if she likes) complete a full circle by returning to face him again.

I call the *Grenoble* position 'the lean back'. You can quite easily get into it from the *Lyon* position. All you have to do is to lean backwards, until your head touches the bed. This should give you very pleasant and unusual sensations, as your partner's penis presses against the *front* of your vagina – and against the famous G-spot.

But do go a bit gently as you lean back, because you are putting your partner's penis under a fair amount of tension. This ought to be very agreeable for him – but a *sudden* lean back could produce pain, and (if you were really violent about it) the ultimate disaster of a ruptured penis. I suppose there are some blokes who *deserve* that sort of thing, but I'm sure you wouldn't want to go to bed with them.

Exotically-minded lovers can find all sorts of variants of the lean back position, by simply trying out the effect of straightening out various legs, and seeing what happens.

Olympique de Paris is a much less ambitious position – and one which is quite easy for most couples, provided the man is moderately supple. First, look back to page 104, and then take up the ordinary female superior *Carcassonne* position described earlier. The man then raises his legs so that his thighs are alongside the woman's bottom. He can then raise them even further so that they're up around her waist – and he can even cross them behind her back.

This is a pleasant, abandoned sort of position, in which the man can repeatedly pull himself up into the woman, creating sensations which both of them will find agreeable.

Biarritz is what might be called the 'Half Cross Bum' position. It's another female superior position – but she turns herself through about 45 degrees on top of the man, a manoeuvre which will give her quite different sensations inside the vagina. This position does give the man a very good opportunity to caress her bottom (and, indeed her breasts if that's what she likes).

The 'Full Cross' or *Vienne* is really just a development of the last one. The woman turns through 90 degrees on top of the man, so that she's lying at right-angles to him. This certainly makes conversation difficult (which is why I give this posture such an abysmally low romance rating), but the effect on the erotic nerve endings can be quite gratifyingly startling.

Face to Face, Sitting

A lot of people like to make love sitting in a chair – though I'd recommend that you choose a nice, comfortable one, which isn't likely to collapse. I'm slightly baffled by books which suggest that couples should make love on deck-chairs; if you try it, do be very careful!

Association Sportive a pleasant face to face sitting position. The bloke sits on a kitchen chair or stool, and the lady just sits astride him, facing him. Some couples like to try out these chair positions first with their clothes on – since they feel that this is rather more risqué. Obviously, the woman just removes her pants and tights – or wears open-crotch ones.

Face to Face Standing

Stade Français involves a couple making love in a standing position, face to face. If you have been making love horizontally in bed for years, and need something new to make sex more varied, then this could be the answer.

Standing sex has had a bit of a bad press – mainly because it tends to be used for illicit love-making by young couples who have no bedroom to go to. But in fact it can be very pleasant.

Since men are usually a bit taller than their female partners its easier if the man can stand so that he's a little *lower* than his partner. If you're both on the same level, it can be a bit of a strain on the legs – and you may well find out why this position is often referred to as the 'dreaded knee-trembler'!

Racing Club is another version of face to face love-making while standing up. The man lifts the woman up so that she can wrap her legs round him. This is a most entertaining position, which tends to appeal to couples with a sense of humour – but it's best not attempted if the man has any back trouble.

Rear Entry

Now we move on to the 'rear entry' positions. Some people don't like these, because they consider them undignified and rather too close to what goes on in the animal world. But some rear entry positions can be very comfortable – particularly the 'Spoons' one, which we'll come to in a moment. Also, some of them are very practical during pregnancy.

Furthermore, these positions can help a lot of women who need extra clitoral stimulation during intercourse. For in a rear-entry position, one great advantage is the fact that it is easy for the man to reach round with his hand and stimulate the woman's clitoris with his fingertips. Quite often, this can help her achieve orgasm during intercourse when otherwise she wouldn't have done so.

Most common rear entry positions are practised with the man above. But it's also perfectly possible to make love rear entry-style with the woman above.

A very similar position, but this time on a chair, is the *Bègles*.

Then there's the 'Spoons' or *Dax* – a comfortable, cosy position. The couple lie on their sides on the bed, with the man snuggled up behind the woman. This is a nice way for a couple to cuddle up together on a cold winter's night – and perhaps fall asleep afterwards, their bodies curving harmoniously together like two spoons in a drawer. (This one is good in pregnancy too.)

Very sensuous are several variations on this theme. The first of these is similar to the Spoons – but with the woman bending the top half of her body right forward until it's at 90 degrees to the man's body. In a second variation, the man leans backwards. And similar to this last one is a third variation, in which the woman thrusts her leg backwards between the man's thighs, as far as it'll go. Surprisingly enough, this produces strikingly different and pleasant sensations.

Finally, one rear entry position which is worth trying is the standing one. The woman can 'develop' this by bending forward, if she wants to. If she's quite lithe and lissom, she may want to experiment with the sensations caused by bending very far forward until her hands touch the floor. Provided your lover isn't the sort of idiot who tries to drive your head through the carpet, this can be very agreeable. Also worth trying is bending forward over a comfortable sofa or armchair.

Q **I am eight months pregnant, but still very much enjoy making love with my husband. Only trouble is, it's getting a bit uncomfortable now, what with my 'bump'!**

Are there any positions which would be more comfortable?

A There are many, ma'am. Probably the most popular for expectant mums is the one in which you simply lie face to face on top of your husband.

This is known in the obstetric world as the 'Mother Superior' position . . .

Q **Re: the position you described as 'having a bit on the side' my husband and I have attempted it, and we think it is impossible.**

A You really must try harder, ma'am! All you have to do is lie on your back with knees raised. Your husband then lies on his side with his thighs curled up under your bottom. I'd come round and demonstrate, but I do not make house calls.

Premature Ejaculation

These days, increasing numbers of women are unwilling to put up with premature ejaculation ('hair-trigger trouble'). And a good thing too, in my opinion!

In the olden days (like about 1960), there was no effective treatment for this all-too-common male condition. Furthermore, women were willing to accept the fact that lots of guys could only 'manage it' for a couple of minutes. But today, it seems to me that the average Britoness demands much, much more! Certainly the latest figures suggest that the late 1980s woman isn't prepared to put up with sexual intercourse lasting only two or three minutes – she frequently prefers 15 or 20 minutes or more. So, if her mate is ejaculating too prematurely for her, she takes him along to the doc for treatment.

Hang on – before we get to treatment, why does premature ejaculation happen at all? Well, it does seem to me that some chaps are by nature rather explosively triggered – especially when they're young. But orthodox teaching says that most prematurely ejaculating males were *conditioned* by their early sexual experiences.

In other words, they first made love in situations, like the back of car, were they felt that they had to reach a climax fast – and they've gone on doing so ever since.

But the great thing is, nowadays you can treat your man's hair-trigger trouble.

For by far the most efficient way of treating 'PE' is the one developed by US sex researchers Johnson and Masters, who found that if a woman uses an 'orgasm delay grip' on her man, she can re-train him over a period of months, so that eventually he can last for as long as they both wish.

The exact explanation of the delay grip must be taught over several weeks by a Johnson and Masters therapist. (Ask your doc to refer you to one.)

The grip – which has to be very precise – involves placing your thumb on one part of your man's penis, and your index and middle fingers on the prescribed location on the opposite side. You then give a deft squeeze and the not-unpleasant sensation which this produces will stop him from reaching a climax.

It's rather like stopping a sneeze by pressing your upper lip – but a good deal more fun.

Q I am married to a dentist who suffers from premature ejaculation. I have tried to put up with this over the years.

Unfortunately, he recently had what he thought was the brilliant idea of using some local anaesthetic ointment on his penis in order to reduce his sensitivity and slow him down. After he'd used it about half a dozen times, I suddenly got an intense redness and soreness of my vaginal opening, which has driven me nearly crazy.

I have been unable to make love at all since then. This is extremely frustrating for me, because in actual fact, what my husband doesn't know is that I have to obtain all of my sexual satisfaction through having an affair with his partner.

A I'm sorry to hear about this dreadful mess. As regular readers of my work will know, most cases of inflammation of the vulva are due to infection.

In case this is so, you should immediately go to a clinic or a doctor who is equipped to make the tests for the common genital infections.

But I suspect that what has happened here is that you've developed a violent 'sensitivity reaction' to your husband's ointment. This is very common with local anaesthetics, and I actually had such a reaction myself once – though only (I hasten to add) through using it for sunburn.

If it is a sensitivity reaction, your doc will probably treat you with anti-histamine pills.

When you've recovered, why don't you and your husband go along to a clinic which specialises in the more sensible way of treating premature ejaculation?

Q I love my fiancé very much, but he 'comes' almost as soon as he gets inside me. This has hit his confidence very badly. We are supposed to get married next year, but I am afraid that if this goes on, he will call everything off.

A Your fiancé is suffering from a very common male complaint called 'premature ejaculation' – which is also known as 'hair trigger trouble.'

There's a simple method of treatment called 'Masters-Johnson therapy.' If you and your chap go together to a Family Planning Clinic, they'll be able to point you in the direction of a therapist who specialises in this kind of problem.

Promiscuity

The fact has to be faced that promiscuous sexual behaviour has now become very widespread in young people – in women as well as in men.

Distinguished British sociologist Michael Schofield studied a large group of 25-year-olds, some of whom were married.

He found that:

almost one third of them had had *no* sex partners in the previous year

almost one third had had only *one* partner in a year

a tiny proportion had had just *two* partners in a year

but a full third had had *three or more* partners (sometimes many more) in the course of a year.

So Schofield found that nowadays a very large proportion of women and men in their early-to-mid twenties do go through a decidedly promiscuous phase. It cannot be denied that the rise in VD in western society – and the emergence of new and alarming types of sexually transmitted disease – is related to the fact that people do have many more partners these days.

Regrettably, there are a lot of men in this age group who have a quite extraordinarily aggressive appetite for sexual conquest, and who will quite cheerfully have sex with 200 partners per year or more, if let loose. Anyone with even a passing acquaintance with bacteriology will realize that this sort of foolish, irresponsible behaviour unfortunately provides a sort of perpetual Christmas party for germs!

Happily, most men and women who go through a rather promiscuous phase between about 20 and 26 do eventually get over it and settle down to a monogamous – or at least relatively monogamous – relationship which they intend to be life-long.

Q I am 26 and thinking of settling down and getting married. But one thing worries me. It's this: I counted up on my fingers the other day and found that I have had no less than 11 lovers. Do you think this makes me terribly promiscuous?

A No – but it does rather sound as if you have 11 fingers. Seriously, people do vary a great deal in the amount of sexual experience they've had. Recently I tried to reassure a woman of about the same age as yourself that it was perfectly normal for her to be a virgin. Similarly, by today's standards it's not very unsual for a 26-year-old to have slept with 11 men over (presumably) quite a few years. You seem to have survived these experiences, and I hope you enjoyed them.

Prostate Gland

The prostate gland is about the size of a chestnut. In fact, if you imagine a conker with a hole through, you'll have a good idea of what a prostate is like.

It's located just below the bladder. The urethra (or urinary pipe) runs straight through it. It's claimed that this makes it the exact embryological equivalent of the Famous Female G-Spot.

What does it *do*? Well, its only known function is a sexual one. It adds a fair old contribution to the fluid which a man ejaculates when he has a climax. The prostatic secretion is thought to give impetus to the sperms in some way – and the added volume probably does give a boost to his sensual satisfaction.

Disorders

There are two main problems with the prostate gland: *enlargement*, and *cancer.*

In most men, the gland increases markedly in size after about the age of 50. For fairly obvious reasons of 'plumbing', this tends to interfere with the water-works. Indeed, if the enlargement is too great, it may become impossible to pass urine.

Prostate trouble is so common that two recent British prime ministers have had theirs removed. As an alternative to removal, there is a newer and milder operation called a 'TUR' in which part of the gland is nibbled away by a slim instrument pushed up the urinary pipe.

Cancer of the prostate is, of course, far more serious. It is treated (often successfully) by removal of the gland, plus hormone therapy and possibly radiation.

Stimulation

From a sexual point of view, prostatic stimulation is possible and (I gather) widely practised in the more exotic parts of the world.

It is done by gentle massage with a well-lubricated finger and tends to produce a more intense climax with a more powerful ejaculation. However, as the massage has to be via the gent's bottom, there are obviously hygenic risks involved.

Q I have blonde hair, which is natural, I might add. But my pubic hair is dark. and my lover wants me to dye it blonde. Would there by any harm in this?

A Well I certainly wouldn't do it because your bloke wants you to do it – only take the plunge if *you* fancy the idea of having blonde pubes.

Tinting your 'maidenhair' involves very little more risk than tinting the hair on your head. However, you should certainly do a test first – and of course drop the whole idea if you develop the slightest soreness or irritation.

But an adverse reaction is most unlikely, and you know what they say: blondes have more fun.

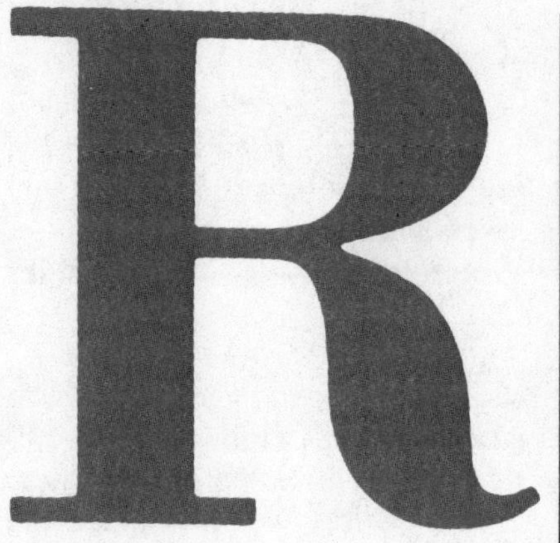

Rape

Rape is a hideous crime. In many cases, it's associated with terrifying violence. Some of the letters I've received in my postbag over the years from women who've been raped make it clear that being the victim of this sort of thing is a shattering experience which leaves the woman feeling dirty, degraded and (perhaps surprisingly) guilty.

And doctors who have treated rape victims are well aware that often they are psychologically scarred for life. Quite often, the ordeal that these women are subjected to is far more brutal and disgusting than you would guess from reading the reports in the newspapers.

Indeed, many cases are *never* reported in the papers – simply because a lot of women never report the attack to the police. This is partly due to a lack of confidence in the way the police will handle the matter.

Alas, it can't be denied that in Britain, Europe and America, police forces have a pretty abysmal record in dealing with women who have reported a rape. However, things *are* slowly improving – partly thanks to the widespread development of Rape Crisis Centres run by women.

Avoiding Rape

Regrettably, no woman is entirely safe from rape – specially as it so often happens within the home. I've tried here to set out some guidelines on how to avoid rape; what to do if somebody attempts it; and what to do afterwards:

1 Don't walk along dark or lonely roads, or cross open ground when there's nobody about.
2 Be particularly wary at night – and especially in the hours after the pubs close (many rapes are alcohol-related).
3 At night, it's far better to take a cab than to walk – the expense may prevent you from having a dangerous experience (or even save your life).
4 Never accept lifts from men – especially late at night.
5 Never travel in single train compartments by yourself – pick an open compartment with other people in it, and sit near another woman.
6 Keep your doors and accessible windows locked, and put a chain on your front door.
7 If you *have* to go out at night, consider carrying a 'rape alarm' – a small canister that gives out a loud and alarming noise.
8 Attend self-defence classes for women.
9 If the law permits it in your country (it doesn't in Britain), consider carrying a weapon for defending yourself.

What to Do if You're Attacked

If a man, or group of men, starts being troublesome, you still have a good chance of avoiding rape. Follow the following rules.

1 At all costs, *don't look submissive* – women's anti-rape groups quite rightly teach that a woman who looks alert and ready to fight back may put the man off.
2 Yell for help – noise is a good deterrent and does actually frighten some men off.
3 Show active resistance: for instance, if a hand is put on you, grab the man's little finger (which is weak) and rip the hand away. Allowing a hand to remain on you will be interpreted as an invitation to go further.
4 If you think you have a reasonable chance of success, *fight back hard* – using any available methods (e.g. kicking him in the testicles, gouging him in the eye, ramming in a high heel or the tip of an umbrella).
5 As an alternative, it may be worth trying to *talk* your way out: some women have succeeded by striking up some sort of brief rap-

port and getting the man to discuss his problems.

6 Don't forget devious ploys like pretending you have womb cancer or VD – these have saved some women in the past.

7 At the point when all seems lost, remember that a man with an erection can be disabled for five or 10 seconds by grasping his organ firmly and twisting it ferociously through about 90°.

8 If you do get free by violent methods, then for heaven's sake, *run*. (Kick off any high heels.) If you're caught again, you're going to get hurt.

9 If you're in fear of your life – e.g. if he has a gun or knife – then *give in*: at least you'll stay alive.

10 Finally, whatever happens, try to fix every detail about the rapist's appearance in your mind.

What to Do if You Have Been Raped

It's a terribly shocking experience, but do your best to follow these guidelines.

1 Get to a phone and ring a Rape Crisis Centre (Rape Control Centre) – these are organizations run by women in many large cities. You'll find the number in the telephone book. Even if the nearest number is far away, ring it (reverse the charges if necessary).

2 Do exactly as the people at the Rape Crisis Centre tell you.

3 Call the police: you may feel very much against the idea – but remember that if they catch the rapist, that should protect other women against his activities for quite a while.

4 *Don't* wash and *don't* change your clothes. If a conviction is to be secured, you'll have to have a forensic examination by a specially qualified doctor – and if you wash or change, the evidence will be gone.

5 Unless you're on the Pill or are otherwise protected against pregnancy, then within 24 hours of the rape make sure you find a doctor who will give you the morning-after Pill to prevent you from conceiving.

6 A week or so after being raped you should for your own protection, go to a doctor for preliminary VD tests (there's no point in going any earlier as the tests couldn't be positive).

7 If you become deeply disturbed as a result of what's happened, do keep in touch with the Rape Crisis Centre (01–837 1600) and don't hesitate to seek psychiatric help and counselling.

Romance

Men in particular are all too likely these days to forget the importance of romance in a relationship. Regrettably, books, films and TV often picture sex as an emotionless business, in which people meet, leap into bed together, have intercourse, smoke a cigarette – and move on!

But real life can't be conducted at that level. We're not machines but deeply complex, emotional creatures who need to be cherished and loved. The man or woman who forgets that fact does so at his or her peril.

Romance, Emotion and Sexuality in Women

As Lord Byron remarked:

'Man's love is of man's life a thing apart,

'Tis woman's whole existence.'

As he implied, men would do well to remember that for a woman, love is usually a far more all-embracing, emotional and even spiritual business than it is for a man. Unfortunately, a man may regard sexual intercourse as far and away the most important aspect of a love relationship with a woman. But it's vital for him to realize that most women see life and love quite differently. A woman is *most* unlikely to view her relationship with a man in crude terms of a penis entering her vagina.

Instead, her view of the love relationship is likely to be bound up with such things as:

the warm glow she feels when he's around

the sense of being valued and wanted as a person by him

the feeling of rightness and completeness that comes from being one half of a loving couple.

If a man doesn't appreciate that his partner has this strongly romantic perception of the love relationship, then he may well be heading for trouble. Certainly, a vast number of marriages founder these days simply because the man fails to satisfy the woman's need for romance.

Romantic Tips for Men

What amazes me after so many years in the advice business is that again and again men go wrong because they fail to follow a few simple 'do's and don'ts'.

Do:

take the trouble to smarten yourself up before you meet her

hold her hand

catch her eye and smile at her when you're in a crowd.

compliment her on her appearance

tell her she smells nice

buy her flowers (they're very inexpensive when you consider what rich dividends they pay!)

take her for candlelit suppers (in all surveys of 'what women consider romantic', dinner by candlelight scores very high).

Don't

ignore her all evening when you're out at a party together

fall in the door after work in the evening and forget to kiss her

flop down in front of the television and forget to talk to her all evening

wander around the bedroom in smelly socks

get into bed unshaven or unwashed

assume that once in bed, you can simply leap on her without any preliminaries

fall asleep the moment you've reached your climax (you could at least say 'Goodnight'!).

Romance, Emotion and Sexuality in Men

The outstanding US expert on sex, Dr Bernie Zilbergeld, neatly encapsulated an all-too-common male view of male sexuality and what man is supposed to contribute to the sex relationship in his famous phrase which describes a man's fantasy-view of his penis: 'two foot long, and hard as steel, and it goes all night . . .'

Of course, this phallic-orientated, male chauvinistic attitude is quite ridiculous! But most men will find echoes of it in the back of their own minds. And it's as well for women to bear in mind that this attitude exists – because it explains many of the stranger aspects of male sexual behaviour!

In particular, it explains why men are so often worried about their phalluses. Most males have worries such as:

is it big enough?

will I be able to get it erect?

how long will I be able to keep it up?

will I be able to get it up *again*?

So if you're a woman, keep in mind the fact that a man's attitude to sex and love is likely to be very genitally orientated.

And if you're a man, just consider whether it wouldn't be better to move away from these old macho ideas. Thank heavens, as we move into the last years of the twentieth century, there's an increasing trend towards the idea of what's been called 'the new man' – the man who's more concerned with being gentle and caring and sharing with his partner than with being obsessed with his own phallus.

But whether he's a 'new man' or the most ghastly of old-style 'macho men', the fact is that he too *probably needs a spot of romance in his love-life*. So I'll conclude this section with a few hints to help women make their partners feel romantic – and loved.

Romantic Tips for Women

Do:

tell him he's handsome – even if he isn't

take the trouble to see to your make-up and hair before you meet him (aggrieved feminists please note: I have given similar advice to *men* elsewhere in this book)

consider turning off the TV and giving him a cuddle instead.

Don't:

(as the song says) 'send him off with your hair all in curlers'

welcome him home with curlers in

wear terrible 'passion-killing' underwear in bed

heave a sigh of resignation as soon as you realize he has love-making in mind

say awful, unromantic things after love-making, like 'Would you please pass me a tissue to clear up this mess?'.

A Lifetime of Romance

Alas, today's fast-increasing trend is for marriages to go on the rocks. It seems to me that the best chance of reversing this alarming drift towards divorce is simply to *bring back romance*.

A ward sister recently told me about an old lady whom she had been nursing. This woman was 87 and had been married for about 60 years – yet before every visiting time she took enormous care to put on an elegant lace gown, make herself up beautifully, and dab a spot of perfume behind her ears.

Why? 'Well,' she told the ward sister, 'my husband is a *very* romantic man, you know . . . '

It gives you fresh hope, doesn't it?

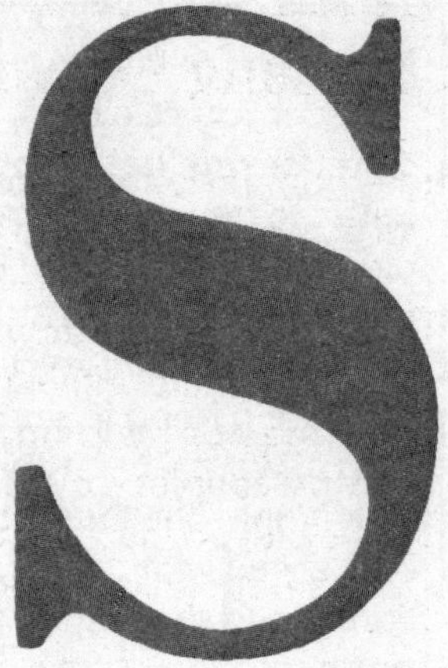

Rubbing Oils

The great US sex researchers Masters and Johnson found that the use of a massage oil was very helpful to couples with sexual difficulties. And of course, masseurs (and masseuses) have known for thousands of years that a body massage is improved by the use of an oil. You too may find a body oil helpful – to rub on the sexual or non-sexual parts of your partner's body, as you choose.

Important considerations are that the oil shouldn't be harmful or irritant to the skin or genitals; that it shouldn't stain the sheets!

Sex shops sell preparations with names like Love Oil, Love Cream, Joy Jelly, and Emotion Lotion! These usually contain perfumes, so there is a small risk of a sensitivity reaction if they are applied to delicate tissues.

In fact, vast numbers of couples in Britain, America and other countries have discovered that equally good results can be achieved by gently anointing each other's bodies with simple products such as baby oil or body lotion. For best results, remember to warm the oil in your hands before rubbing it into your loved one's shoulders, arms or whererever.

Settling Down

Perhaps fortunately for the future of humanity, the great majority of women and men regard it as desirable to settle down with one partner for life, either in marriage or by living together.

Most couples – even those who have played the field for some years – are only too glad to settle into a mutual loving relationship in which they devote themselves to each other permanently – and have sex only with each other.

How often should they have sex? I wish I had a pound for every time somebody has written in asking me this question! The answer is that there are no very definite rules.

Dr Kinsey was the first to establish that the 'average' couple made love 2.4 times a week. At the beginning of 'settling down', couples tend to make love a little more often than this but later it's a little less. Other surveys over the last 40 years or so have confirmed that he was roughly right. But the important thing to realize is that as long as *both* partners are happy, it doesn't matter how often they make love.

The real problem arises when (as is so often the case) one partner wants to have sex frequently, while the other doesn't. This often happens, and when a woman who likes intercourse four times a week marries a man who only likes it once a month (or, indeed, *vice versa*), then trouble is brewing! Indeed, under these circumstances it's quite unusual for the marriage to survive. It is therefore important to try to marry somebody with more or less the same amount of interest in sex.

Q I am extremely passionate in mid-cycle, but then my sex drive vanishes. Round about ovulation, my sexual instincts are at full steam, and I lust after my husband.

Then after I've tired him out – that's it for the rest of the month. Can I do anything about this?

A Well, some women are like you. P'raps it's nature's way of ensuring that sex is most likely when you're at your most fertile.

However, two possibilities do occur to me. Firstly you may be losing interest in the second half of the cycle because of some sort of 'pre-menstrual syndrome'. If so, your doc might be willing to consider hormone treatment – e.g. with the dreaded progesterone suppositoires. And, second like some women, you may have a deeper feeling that sex should only be enjoyable when conception is possible. Psychotherpy could help this.

If neither of these suggestions is correct then just be happy that you're having a great time in the middle of the month.

Q My husband enjoys playing sex games during our love-making. If I say that I find them disgusting, he gets very upset and says it must be that I don't love him.

For instance, he wants to rub fruit-flavoured gel onto our bodies so that we can lick it off afterwards.

How can I get it through to him, without upsetting him, that these things are a turn off for me?

A Difficult, ma'am. People have wildly differing views on what is exciting, and what is disgusting in the bedroom.

My feeling is that you ought to be utterly frank and honest: write down a list of sex practices that you find repellent, hand it to him and say that – as much as you love him – you wouldn't want to do these with *anybody*.

If he takes that personally, then I'm afraid that's his problem.

Incidentally, re the 'fruit flavoured gel' which you find distasteful: it might just be worth trying fruit-flavoured 'Booby-Drops'. Since these are designer-made for love-making, they could be more aesthetically acceptable to you.

Q My husband wants to kiss my bottom intimately. Is this wise?

A No. Anilingus, or anilinctus, as it is also called, is thought to be responsible for the very high incidence of hepatitis in male homosexuals.

Q My fiancé wants me to use cocaine with him, and says it will improve our sexual satisfaction. What do you think?

A I think he's crazy. He'll probably end up impotent – and *you'll* probably end up in jail or in the cemetery (neither of which places is particularly noted for sexual satisfaction).

Q I would do almost anything sexually to keep my man, but now he's got this persistent kinky idea that he wants to urinate inside me.

A Well, don't let him! I get quite a few letters about various urinary games. Some are fairly harmless, but I reckon this one could damage your delicate vaginal tissues. Next time he asks, tell him to p . . . off.

Q My husband and I have always had a romantic desire to make love in the sea.

But when we tried last summer we weren't able to manage it. I just couldn't seem to get him in.

Why? Is it something to do with sea water?

A Yes, although making love in the briny sounds very romantic, it can be quite tricky – especially if there are sharks about!

More seriously, there are two basic problems. One is that you may be a bit tensed up, particularly if you're afraid that you might be spotted by someone on a passing pedalo.

Secondly, the sea does tend to instantly wash away the feminine 'love juices' which are so essential for an amatory encounter. (NB This is why mermaids are so unsuccessful in reproducing – or so I believe.)

Anyway, the answer to all this is to use a simple water-stable vaginal lubricant – the type you can buy without embarrassment at any British chemist's.

This year, pack a tube without fail. Happy holidays!

Q My boyfriend is heavily into books like *The Story of* O and the works of the Marquis de Sade. He's obsessed with wanting to stick objects up my backside. Now he wants me to get engaged. Do you think I should!

A No! Anyone who has the bad taste to read boring books like *The Story of* O (which, despite its prominent place on station bookstalls, is only marginally less tedious than the works of the Marquis de Sade) is really not worth getting engaged to.

As to his sexual proclivities, he's clearly a nut, and you would be well-advised to drop him. I should tell him what to do with his engagement ring. But watch out – in view of his tastes, he'll probably take you literally!

Q My husband has been reading a lot of sex manuals and has decided to buy me something called a 'clitoris stimulator' for my birthday. Could you please explain what on earth this is?

A Well ma'am, it's a device which is intended to do what it says – that is stimulate your clitoris. Basically it's a little ring which fits around the base of your man's penis. On top of the ring is a protruberance with various bumps or ridges on it.

The general idea is that these are supposed to rub against your clitoris while your bloke is making love to you. In practice, the device doesn't work very well, and can slip sideways and give you a nasty poke in the groin. Happy Birthday!

Q My husband likes me to go out in the evening wearing no knickers. How would you view this?

A By lying on the floor, I suppose! Seriously, this is an increasingly common habit among women – mainly for health reasons. Wearing no knickers may be a bit draughty, but it probably does help to protect you against thrush and other common vaginal problems.

Q I read the best-seller *Lace* by Shirley Conran, and was surprised by the scene in which the Arab prince puts a wriggling goldfish into the heroine's vagina, in order to stimulate her. What would really happen if one did this?

A I don't think it would be very nice – particularly for the goldfish. Honestly, I think authors just stick these scenes into novels to make a sensation (Shirley Conran certainly achieved worldwide publicity with *that* particular idea).

I've never encountered anybody who was daft enought to use a goldfish as a vibrator – and I hope I never do.

Q My boyfriend wants to make love to me in his whirlpool bath. Are there any gynaecological risks in this?

A Well, you could get pregnant. To be serious, the main risks of whirlpool baths arise if they're used by a lot of people. Thus, public and hotel tubs have been incriminated in outbreaks of skin rashes and sore eyes. Also, in America some 14 members of a women's racquet-ball team went in a whirlpool bath together, and caught legionnaires disease.

Q My fiancé and I are going to the States later this year, and he is quite determined that on the flight we should join the 'Mile High Club'.

I understand that you 'join' it by making love in an aeroplane when it is more than a mile up.

I was a bit doubtful initially, but I must say it sounds quite exciting. However, could we get into trouble? And would the lack of air pressure do me any harm?

A This is definitely rather naughty behaviour, you know. However, the 'Mile High Club' does exist, and I am told that many of its members are airline staff, for obvious reasons.

But please bear in mind the practicalities. It is very difficult to make love on an aeroplane seat (or seats) unless the plane is virtually deserted. The alternative – which, I believe, is how many members of the Club qualified – is to make love in the loo. That sounds a teeny bit sordid to me – and also *very* cramped. (You could get yourself caught on the soap dispenser.)

Now I'm told that the airlines don't often prosecute anybody for engaging in this unusual form of 'in-flight entertainment.' But it would be awfully embarrassing if you were caught.

On the other hand, they can hardly chuck you out! And, to answer your final query, there are no physiological ill-effects associated with making love in the sky, no matter how high you go.

Q My wife wants to make love in a sauna. I suppose this is all a very romantic, but is it technically possible? Surely the wooden seats would be far too hot for a couple to lie down on?

A I'm sorry it's taken some time to answer your question, sir – but it has required a bit of research in Finland and elsewhere.

Love-making in the sauna is frowned on by the Finns (and, indeed, by Haringey Borough Council). But it is, in fact, technically possible, and quite often practised in Nordic lands.

You'll recall that in the traditional Finnish sauna there are usually three levels of benches (or *lauteet*). Apparently, the simplest method of love-making is for the *nainen* (or female partner) to sit on the second level of *lauteet* facing forwards. The *mies* (or male partner) then stands on the tiled floor in front of her and embraces her – taking care not to get overheated in the *löyly* (or steam). What all this does to the *verenpaine* (or blood pressure), I do not know. But afterwards, they both go off for a cold shower – or else jump in the lake.

Q My husband invariably wants to make love to the sound of symphonic music. Is this unusual?

A Not at all, ma'am! In fact, I'd strongly recommend Brahm's First, Beethoven's Fifth, and Berlioz's *Fantastic*.

But think twice about Tchaikovsky's *Pathetique* and Schubert's *Unfinished*...

Q My husband read *Fear of Flying* by Erica Jong, in which the heroine brings another woman to a climax with a champagne bottle. Now he wants to do the same thing to me.

A A naff idea, ma'am. Very few things should be poked up the vagina, apart from the structure which nature, through some miracle, designed to fit it so perfectly.

Many couples who go in for these penetrative vaginal games don't realise that a woman's tissues are delicate, and tear easily.

Furthermore the magazine, *World Medicine* reported a case in which a Cumbrian couple tried to use a bottle of Bollinger as a dildo. Three months later, the cork had to be surgically removed...

Q My husband is always thinking up romantic and sexy things to do to me. But is his latest idea safe? He wants to bring home flowers, and use them to 'decorate' the various openings of my body.

A Well, if he only wants to stick a hibiscus blossom (*without* stem) in your ear, that's OK.

But pushing floral tributes up people's naughty bits is really not on! It can lead to infection, or damage delicate tissues.

Indeed, I remember a young bridegroom whom we had to operate on to remove the carnation stem which his 'stag night' pals had unwisely jammed into a very unfortunate place!

Sexual Fantasy

I'm always entertained by those mysterious small ads for 'rainwear' which appear in the most respectable newspapers. In case you don't know, these adverts are keenly perused by a very large number of people who – for some reason – are into making love with each other in plastic macs!

I suppose one shouldn't really make fun of other people's sexual habits. But I'm only poking *gentle* fun, especially as the 'rainwear lovers' do at least have the merit of being totally harmless to anyone else

Anyway, this month I'm intrigued to find out that worldwide there are now so many of them they've actually formed an international society, with its own quarterly journal, giving hints on rainwear fashions, plus details of barbecues, social evenings, and heaven knows what else.

It's called *La Société Mackintosh Internationale* (or if you're German, *Die Internationale Mackintosh Gesellschaft*).

If any readers are into that sort of thing, then as the *Société's* brochure says:

Pourquoi ne pas vous informer avec plus de détails . . . vous n'avez qu'à envoyer une enveloppe addressée à vous-même, avec un timbre postal, a l'addresse suivante: La Société Mackintosh Internationale, PO Box No 33, Horley, Surrey RH6 8NB.

Q My boyfriend wants to have intercourse with him while we are ice-skating. Is this really possible?

A Sounds chilly, and liable to get you arrested. But there are certain Torville-and-Dean-type poses in which it would be distinctly possible.

However, don't fall over – or you may discover a new definition of the word frigidity . . .

Q I am having a lot of trouble with two men in my office. They pinch my bottom and make offensive remarks about my breasts. Any suggestions?

A It's become increasingly clear in recent years that a lot of women are justifiably very upset by this tedious kind of sexual harassment at work.

Anyone who is subjected to attentions which she resents should consider these guidelines:

object *at once* – if you let things go on, they may get worse

if you belong to a union, complain at once – preferably to a female official

talk to other women at work about the problem

if necessary, tell the man that you'll complain to higher authority about his behaviour

if he *is* 'higher authority', then consider whether it's worth going to a lawyer – or the police.

if nothing can be done, don't stay in a job where you're miserable – leave

While I'm on the subject of sexual harassment at work, could I draw attention to one particularly dreadful manifestation of it?

Ever since I qualified in the early 60s, I've come across cases where lunatics working in factories have thought it a 'great joke' to put a high-pressure air hose up colleagues' skirts. *If the compressed air enters the victim's body (through the vagina or rectum), terrible damage can be done.*

Just before I wrote this book, yet another case of this form of harassment came before the courts. The woman victim escaped with her life, but was left with a permanent colostomy. I hope the man who did it is pleased with himself.

Q I am very surprised by what appears to be a new trend in sexual behaviour. These days, whenever we invite some couple over, the husband seems to go out of his way to catch me alone after dinner in the kitchen and grope me. Is this considered 'socially acceptable' today, or what?

A Well now you come to mention it, it does seem to me that these days the social after-dinner goodnight kiss has been widely replaced by the social after-dinner goodnight grope. All kinds of blokes, appear to think that if they're invited somewhere to dinner, this means that they're entitled to a bit of a cuddle with the hostess afterwards.

I suppose this doesn't matter very much if the hostess is keen on that sort of thing. But sexual harassment is *never* justifiable – even in the erotic post-prandial atmosphere so often induced by good food and good wine.

So cooks (of whichever sex) be careful whom you invite into the kitchen to help with the washing-up. If in doubt, hit'em with your wok.

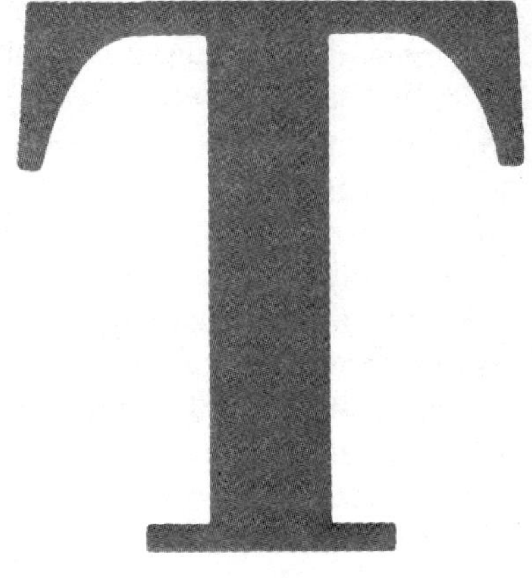

The Testicle

It is fairly important for a woman to have a working knowledge of the male testicle – if only because it's so awfully easy for her to damage it in bed!

All too commonly, a swiftly-raised feminine knee catches a chap in the wrong place, and immediately deprives him of the power of speech (not to mention anything else) for quite a while.

Happily, the pain and shock is as a rule only temporary, and I have not known any gent to suffer permanent harm or infertility as a result of such a bedtime accident.

But the testicle (also known as the testis, or 'ball'), is an incredibly pain sensitive part of the male body. This fact is vital to remember if you're attacked by a man. If at all possible, smash him as hard as you can in the testicles with knee, foot, fist, umbrella or whatever – and then run like hell, because (as I say) the disability is only temporary!

Turning to happier topics, the testicle is of course the source of the millions of sperms whose aim in life is to unite with a ripe ovum from your ovary and so form a baby.

The sperms which are produced by the testicle find their

way up through a man's 'plumbing', in order to be ejaculated at the moment of climax. Anything up to 500 million of these crafty little rascals are produced in a single orgasm.

The two testicles have another function, which is to produce the male sex hormones, which give a lad his secondary male sex characteristics of hairiness muscularity, stroppiness, aggressive driving, and so on.

Each testicle is rather like a flattened ping-pong ball in shape and size. Average dimensions are about one and three quarter inches long, one and a quarter inches deep, and one inch thick.

Blokes are always worrying about the size of their testicles, but the actual dimensions matter little, provided the things work all right. If a man appears to be firing on both cylinders, then he needn't worry.

It's quite common for one testis to be slightly smaller than the other, and this too is quite normal. In virtually all men, one orb hangs slightly lower than the other but the reason for this is not known. A curious property of the testis is that it will retract rapidly upwards if it's threatened in any way. Try poking the inside of your man's thigh with a pencil and you'll see what I mean!

Testicles occasionally have to be removed because of accident or disease. Happily, these days it's possible to replace a lost testis with a plastic one which feels like the real thing.

Q If I refuse to let my fiancé make love to me, he complains that he gets an extremely intense pain in he testicles. Isn't he making all this up?

A Nope. If a bloke is sexually excited by kissing and cuddling but doesn't get the chance to reach a climax, he very often *does* get pain in his testicles.

This common ache is known as 'the gravels' or 'lover's nuts'. But my friend and colleague Dr Richard Gordon (remember *Doctor In The House?*) long ago christened it with the rather more elegant appellation of *orchitis amorosa acuta*.

Some women get a similar ache – possibly originating in their ovaries – when they've been stimulated but deprived of reaching an orgasm. So quite seriously, this 'frustration pain' is pretty widespread in both sexes.

The cure, I'm afraid, is still to come.

Troilism

This is an activity, common in some quarters, in which three people go to bed together. I make no moral comment on this, because that's not my brief. It's clear the troilism appeals to a lot of people for a variety of reasons. There are two types:

The Two Women in Bed with One Man Situation

This appeals to most males' sexual fantasies of course – since studies show that secretly, most men are very attracted by the idea of going to bed with as many women as possible – 50 or 100 perhaps. Girlie magazines encourage this sort of fantasy with the more girls the merrier, all of them eager to be satisfied! In reality, this wouldn't do the man a lot of good, since one man usually has enough trouble satisfying *one* woman – let alone two (or 100!).

It's also a little difficult to see what the two women are supposed to get out of this kind of troilism, unless, they have lesbian tendencies. My suspicion – based on talking to a number of people who've gone in for troilism – is that what the girls usually get out of it is *money*.

The Two Men in Bed with One Women Situation

As far as I can make out, this definitely does have an appeal for some women (though emphatically *not* for most) because of the higher chance of sexual satisfaction – and the feeling of being admired and wanted by not just one man, but two.

Why this situation appeals to some *men* isn't entirely clear. But there does seem to be a tendency for some men to feel their own sexual efforts to satisfy their partners aren't really sufficient, and should be augmented by those of good old Charlie down the road.

I have to say that I think there's a very real danger that if good old Charlie is any use in bed, he might end up going off with the woman (or, for all I know, with the other man!).

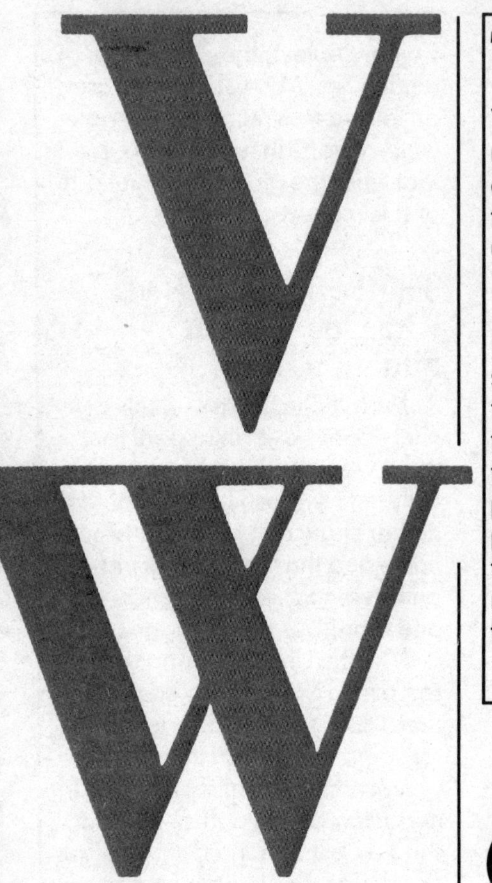

The Vagina

Your vagina is one of the most marvellously-designed structures on Earth. Yet the amazing thing is that so many women are brought up to believe that the vagina is 'nasty', 'dirty', or 'not nice'.

In fact, it's none of these things. It's a warm, pink, well-cushioned sheath which is perfect for its intended function in life. That function – let's not mince words – is to fit snugly and lovingly round the penis, so that the sperms are deposited in the right place, and so that both partners derive the maximum possible enjoyment from the act of love.

Regrettably, a lot of people

Q I am a 52-year-old woman. After many years of celibacy, I've started a wonderful relationship with a young man. The only problem is that I am distressingly sore and dry during love-making. Why?

A It's probably a minor hormone deficiency – common in the over-50s. To begin with, try using a lubricant such as KY Jelly or Durol –

don't realize that the vagina is such a capacious and comfortably-upholstered channel. Instead they think it's a very tight passage, up which a man's penis can only be forced with difficulty and with pain.

This is nonsense. In reality, there's a vast amount of room inside the vagina. It 'balloons out' and lengthens quite dramatically during sexual excitement.

When you come to think of it, the vagina *has* to be a pretty distensible organ, because it must be able to dilate widely enough to let a baby's head through.

But, in addition to being remarkably distensible, it can also contract down, particularly at orgasm, to fit perfectly around the penis.

The other thing which the vagina can do is to produce the 'love juices' – the erotically-induced secretions which lubricate the movements of intercourse.

With their bizarre intra-vaginal camera, the US sex researchers Masters and Johnson have shown that when a woman becomes sexually aroused, it's the walls of her vagina which suddenly start pouring out the love juices.

All in all then, ladies, that's a beautiful and a marvellously efficient structure that you've got there.

buyable without embarrassment at any large chemist's. If that fails, ask your doc about hormone creams.

Q My first baby is now five months old. Since she was born, I have lost all my libido, and my vagina is very dry during love-making.

A This is very common, ma'am. The cause if probably to do with the sudden drop in hormones after a baby is born, though it could simply be due to lack of sleep or breastfeeding.

Unfortunately, we haven't come up with any very effective way of treating the lack of libido. But it *does* nearly always go away in the fullness of time. If not, go to a Family Planning Clinic for help.

Getting round the problem of vaginal dryness, however, is quite simple and a lubricant like Durol or KY would probably make life easier for both of you.

Vaginal Dryness

I recently picked up a French women's magazine, whose cover bore a picture of a rather worried looking model, plus the caption *'Madame – avez-vous la SV?'*

Opening the mag, I rapidly found that the mysterious letters 'SV' stood for *'sécheresse vaginale'* – vaginal dryness.

Complaints of vaginal dryness are very common in the UK, France and doubtless most other countries in the world – because dryness makes it very difficult for a woman to have intercourse.

And even if she can just about manage it, it's likely to be at best unenjoyable, and at worst very sore and painful. (It often makes her bloke very red and sore too!)

So why does *'la SV'* occur?

Well, it's not usually due to any physical disorder, except in the case of women who've passed the menopause.

The latter do very often get distressing dryness, due to the fall in their female hormone levels. Happily, this can usually be put right by either: (a) taking female hormone tablets prescribed by a doc; or (b) using a female hormonal vaginal cream (also prescription only).

But among the rest of the female population, vaginal dryness isn't usually a disease or disorder or deficiency.

It's a failure of your 'love juice glands' to lubricate, for two possible reasons: (a) because your man hasn't stimulated you enough by love play;
(b) because you're not relaxed enough.

Obviously, the two things often go together. Problem (a) can be overcome by insisting that your man learns and uses the basic techniques of foreplay. Problem (b) can be difficult, except where there is some clear-cut reason for your tension – for instance a recent episiotomy, or a recent vaginal infection.

Usually the best thing in severe cases is to see a woman doctor at a Family Planning Clinic for a spot of counselling plus vaginal relaxation exercises.

But in the many milder cases, things usually turn out OK if you use a bland vaginal lubricant for a while. KY Jelly is the traditional one, and another fluid one is called Senselle. Both can be bought cheaply over the counter, and you can apply them to your chap as well as yourself.

It used to be thought that the pill caused vaginal dryness, but this now seems unlikely.

Q I am a very lucky girl with a loving, caring, desirable boyfriend. Only problem: I get so sore when we make love that we have to abandon it after a few minutes. Can you help? My boyfriend is not unduly large. And I don't think it's a 'love juice' problem.

A Well, I rather suspect it is, and I think things will get better over the years as you relax – and produce more juices.

But in the meantime, you should go to any chemist and buy a lubricant which will 'ease the passage'.

If they don't work, you and your chap should go to a Family Planning Clinic for technical advice.

Q My vagina is now so loose that I thought my husband would seek sex elsewhere. In order to tighten things up, I have been putting a tampon up my bottom before sex. Is this wise?

A I don't think it's a good idea, ma'am. Sorry to hear about your problems, but I suggest you see a gynaecologist to discuss a tightening up operation.

Vaginal Slackness

So many readers have written in asking where they could buy devices which help improve women's pelvic muscle tone, when the vagina has become slack after having children that I thought I'd better print full details. Perhaps one of the following would make a nice Christmas present!

Anyway, the most sensible vaginal muscle developer seems to me to be the 'Femtone', which is available for £15 (including p & p) from Aleph One Ltd, *The Old Courthouse, Bottisham, Cambridgeshire CB5 9BA*.

The same firm also supply the extraordinary biofeedback perineometer (!), which enables you to play back you vaginal contractions on a loudspeaker, if you fancy that sort of thing! But it does cost a hefty 500 quid!

An alternative is to buy the naughty 'Geisha Balls' or 'Duo Balls'. They are available at any sex shop for a few pounds, and can be 'worn' all day.

Those who use them to develop their vagina muscles say that they're *wickedly* agreeable to use – but they do tend to produce a loud 'clonking' sound as you walk about, which may be a mite embarrassing . . .

Flexing Your Vaginal Muscles

The vaginal muscles form the front part of the pelvic floor muscles – which make up a sort of 'diaphragm' stretched across the lower part of your body.

Now these muscles make a ring round the opening of your vagina, so that they gently grip your man's penis when you are making love with him.

Unfortunately, in quite a lot of women these vaginal muscles go into an involuntary spasm whenever any approach is made to their vaginas. This is the all-to-common condition of 'vaginismus', which makes intercourse painful or down-right impossible.

It is claimed that violent spasm of these vaginal muscles is the cause of rare cases of *penis captivus*. This is the alleged syndrome in which the man becomes trapped inside the woman and cannot withdraw.

Anyway, how do you flex your vaginal muscles?

Quite simple, really. Next time you are making love, just 'twitch' the lower front part of your body, as if you were trying to stop yourself from spending a penny.

Your man will immediately feel a gentle but pleasant squeezing sensation. Indeed, it may be that as a result he will immediately reach an unwanted early climax, and spend the rest of the evening cursing me! So perhaps you'd better warn him first.

What I have described is actually the first of the two 'Kegel exercises', which strengthen a woman's muscles, and help her to avoid prolapse in later life.

You can also use the second Kegel exercise during love-making. This involves tightening up the muscles a little further back (again, with a bit of a 'twitch') as if you were trying to prevent a bowel action. This also produces a gentle vaginal squeeze – which may be perceived by the man as being a little deeper inside.

There are those who claim that after months of practice on these two exercises, a determined woman can acquire such yoga-like control of her vagina muscles that she can use the outer and inner muscles alternately.

If this is true (and it may be so), she would presumably emulate the young lady of Brussels –

Whose pride was her vaginal
muscles;
She could easily plex them,
And so interfex them
As to whistle love songs through
her bustles!

Q We are 20 lovely and loving ladies from Farnham, Surrey, and we disagree with your theory about penis size and vaginal soreness.

You said that the woman who thought her boyfriend's penis was too large for her (because she could not have sex with him) was probably wrong – and just suffering from *vaginismus* (vaginal muscle spasm).

Well, some of the 20 ladies in our office have had experiences similar to that described in the reader's letter. And in no case had it anything to do with *vaginismus,* since everything was OK with subsequent partners. You clearly are misinformed!

A Dear lovely (and loving) ladies: we are slightly at cross-purposes here.

Most women have had the experience of being unable to make love with a particular bloke because of one or more of the following factors:

he was too clumsy

he tried to get in before she was ready

she was tensed up

she had some painful vaginal infection (such as thrush)

she'd recently had an episiotomy, or a birth-tear, stitched up

All of these factors are liable to cause intense pain. And quite understandably, that pain frequently produces a terrific 'tightening up' of the vaginal muscles. *That is how* vaginismus *begins*.

With tenderness and commonsense on the part of both partners, the vaginal spasm should go away quite soon – though occasionally it takes months or years.

I repeat that is very, very rare for a couple to find that the man's penis is so big that it genuinely will not go into the vagina.

PS Sorry I had to cut your letter down. It was too long to fit in (if you'll forgive the phrase)!

Q Recently I met a man whom I would like to marry. But the first time we made love left me with considerable soreness next day. And on the next occasion, it was quite impossible.

Since then, a friend has told me that some couples simply cannot make love because the man's penis is too big or the wrong shape. Is this right?

A Such cases are so very, rare that I've never seen one in my life.

What's far more likely is this. You

were able to achieve intercourse the first time, but (for some reason which a doctor would need to sort out) this caused soreness the following day.

Such soreness is often the trigger for the very common condition called **vaginismus** (vaginal muscle spasm) The pain tends to make intercourse difficult or impossible.

So what you need to do now is to go along to an experienced woman doctor at a Family Planning Clinic. She'll examine you and (I hope) teach you the simple techniques of relaxation which will enable you to have painless lovemaking with your man.

Q I'm a girl in my late teens and my very embarrassing problem is (as my friends so delicately phrase it) 'fanny farting'!

Please don't laugh at me. I have only had intercourse with one partner in the past, and I found that when his penis was thrust into my vagina, it seemed to drive in air, compress it, and then push it out, so creating this ghastly noise.

I feel quite anxious about it at the moment, because of the fact that a new, close relationship with a man looks as though it's shortly going to become enhanced into a physical one (Hopefully!).

PS I think your column is ace!

Vaginismus

PAINFUL intercourse (and even complete inability to have intercourse) is frequently caused by vaginismus.

This is a disabling, involuntary spasm of the muscles which form a ring round the vagina, and comes on whenever a woman is sexually approached.

So if you suffer from vaginismus, you'll doubtless have found that if a man tries to make love to you, the muscles of your vagina close in, like a mouth saying 'No' – and also that your thigh and tummy muscles tend to tighten up at the same time, to protect your vaginal area.

If you have vaginismus quite badly, then you won't even be able to tolerate petting – because your body will tense and curl up self-protectively as soon as a man puts his hand anywhere near your thighs.

A Thank you so much – us gents do always appreciate complimentary remarks about our columns.

Now let's be quite serious about this problem of 'vaginal wind'. Long ago, I wrote about this com-

In a minority of cases, it's sparked off by some painful vaginal condition – like a bad attack of thrush, or an extremely tender episiotomy scar (caused by stitches after childbirth). An attempt at intercourse leads to intense pain; this produces muscle spasm which continues for some months. Because of the spasm, the next attempt causes more pain – and so on.

But in most women with vaginismus, there isn't a physical cause. The difficulty is an emotional one though its not intentional (something which men find very difficult to understand!). You see, even today, large numbers of women grow up with the belief that any kind of penetration of the vagina is very dangerous. Characteristically, they are terrified of using tampons. They also react very evasively or angrily if a doctor wants to do a vaginal examination. (Quite often, the doc makes the big mistake of reacting angrily too – and this may foul up their relationship.)

So, a woman who has vaginismus will have great difficulty in relaxing sufficiently to allow intercourse. She may even be a 'virgin wife'.

Happily, women doctors – mostly working in Family Planning Clinics – have developed a form of psychotherapy (Combined with yoga-like exercises) which enables a vaginismal woman to gain control over her muscles. Countless, women have had their sex lives revolutionised through this method. If you have problems with vaginismus, ask your local Family Planning Clinic if they have a woman doctor practising this form of therapy. If they haven't then write (enclosing sae) to the Institute of Psychosexual Medicine, *11 Chandos St, London W1M 9DE.*

mon difficulty in **SHE**. In my lofty medical arrogance, I declared that it only affected women whose vaginas were too lax because of child-bearing.

How wrong I was! I was nearly blown away by a great blast of letters from women who had no babies at all – but were plagued by the same noisome problem.

I've often told that story at medical meetings – just to show how wrong us docs can be. But unfortunately, *at none of these meetings has any doctor been able to suggest a cure for this vaginal flatulence*.

The best I can suggest is that you

use a vaginal aerosol-foam contraceptive, such as Emko or Delfen (no relation!), to try and 'soak up' the air which has been forced into your vagina.

But what if this doesn't work? Well, just bear in mind that it takes *two* to cause this compression of air; in other words, it's the bloke's problem as well as yours, because he's the one that's pushing it in!

So if it happens with your new lover (and it may not), just say 'Ooops – you've driven some air into me with that great piston of yours!'

If he doesnt laugh at *that*, he's probably not worth going to bed with.

Q My husband is thinking of having a vasectomy, but what we do not understand is this: would he still produce the fluid after the operation?

A Vasectomy has become fantastically popular this last year or so – a fact which has enabled many a surgeon to re-furnish the

The Vas Deferens

Here's an important organ which is not very well known to the public. It's the vas deferens – more commonly referred to as 'the vas' (usually pronounced 'vass', rhyming with 'lass'). 'Vas' is Latin for 'vessel', and 'deferens' means 'bringing'. And the vas deferens is the tube which brings sperm up from the testicle towards the penis.

A man normally has two of these tubes; a few men have three, but this is not an advantage to them as we shall see. The vas looks very like a thin piece of spaghetti. It can be felt with the fingertips through the skin of a man's scrotum as it runs up towards the groin.

The reason why there is such a lot of interest in the vas these days is that *it is the bit that is cut in a vasectomy*. Vasectomy just means 'cutting through the vas'.

This popular operation (well over a hundred thousand are being done world-wide every year) just involves making two tiny incisions in the skin of the scrotum, working through them to cut through each vas and tying the ends.

Why are men who have a *third* vas at a disadvantage? Because the surgeon probably will not realize they have an extra vas front room. Lots of couples ask this question – and the answer is that the man *does* continue to produce fluid in exactly the same way as before at his climax. This is because the sperms are so tiny that their absence makes practically no difference at all to its volume.

Q I am embarrassed to say that because my husband's love-making does not entirely satisfy me, I usually bring myself to a climax afterwards with a vibrator.

deferens, and will fail to cut it. In such cases, the vasectomy won't work! However, the sperm test which is done a couple of months or so after a vasectomy will detect the fact that there is another vas deferens, still sending up vast supplies of spermatozoa. The third vas can them be cut and tied off too.

The vas deferens does *not* seem to have any hormonal function. So, cutting through it dosen't interfere with a man's production of sex hormones, or with his virility. It just gives him a great feeling of coinfidence that he is no longer exposing his female partner to the risk of unwanted pregnancy.

My problem is this. We're going abroad on a business trip soon, and I wonder if I could get into difficulties if the customs found the device in my luggage?

A Within Western Europe and North America, customs officers have been fairly used to vibrators. But you might risk confiscation and public embarrassment if you tried to import one into certain Middle Eastern countries. Also, I suggest you take the batteries out: I've heard of one going off in a plane and causing a bomb alert.

Q Much to my alarm, I have found that recently my wife has been doing something rather unusual at the end of intercourse. After I have 'finished' she produces a vibrator and used it to bring herself to her climax. Is this abnormal?

A Well sir, it's increasingly common these days. Most women do *not* regularly reach a climax during intercourse. I don't think it's unreasonable for a woman who is still unsatisfied after her man's orgasm to decide to take matters into her own hands (so to speak).

Not all men can cope with this recent trend in female sexuality. But

I think you should curb your 'alarm' – and just be glad that your missus has found a way of giving herself a buzz . . .

Q I have decided that it would be fun to buy a vibrator for me and my husband to use. But I really don't want to go in one of those dreadful sex shops, so where could I get one?

A Many readers will throw up their hands in horror at the idea of a woman wanting to buy a vibrator. When these devices first came on to the market, I used to think they

Vibrators

Vibrators have been the one really big success of the sex aid industry. Much to my initial surprise, I've had many letters from women who have found them useful in overcoming lack of libido and failure to reach a climax.

The very idea of a vibrator puts many people off to begin with. But a considerable number of patients actually discover that they like them. They seem to be particularly helpful to three groups of females:

women who are on their own (either temporarily or permanently)

women whose husbands are unable to stimulate them properly because of disability (e.g. arthritis)

women whose partners are – to be blunt – not all that skilled at, or enthusiastic about, love-play.

In addition, quite a lot of couples just use vibrators for sheer fun – or perhaps to spare them a lot of effort when they're tired. (One woman told me quite frankly that when her husband was exhausted, they were both more than happy for her to 'finish herself off' with a vibrator.)

The usual thing is for one or other partner just to hold them gently near or on the woman's clitoris, and let the gentle 'buzzing' motion have its effect.

As you'll discover, some vibrators are actually penis-shaped, and can be placed in the vagina. I suspect that these were invented by men; they certainly don't seem to be as popular with women as the clitoral vibrators.

If you do decide to put a vibrator inside the vagina, you should:

were quite crazy – but eventually I realised that a vast number of women (and some men) do find them fun to use in bed. They can also be helpful for sexual problems.

Now, I quite understand your reluctance to visit some sleazy sex shop to buy a vibrator – but you don't have to these days.

Perfectly reputable chain stores do now sell 'electrical massagers' or 'beauty massagers' which work admirably as vibrators. My researchers indicate that many women buy them without embarrassment as 'beauty aids'.

For instance, the Clairol Beauty Massage system (around £9.95 at large chemists) can be used successfully to put a little extra voltage

make absolutely sure that the device is clean

make certain that there are no rough or jagged bits which could hurt

insert *very* gently, perhaps using a lubricant.

Most vibrators are battery-powered, but there are also mains-powered, vibrators. Interestingly these devices are now sold on a massive scale all over the western world in pharmacies and electrical goods shops (rather than sex shops) as 'massagers'.

Ostensibly, they are supposed to be either for 'beauty' or for 'rheumatism' – take your pick! – but it's well known that a vast number of women use the mains-powered massagers for sexual pleasure or relief.

Finally, two words of warning about vibrators – one serious and one not so serious. Firstly, there's a disturbing tendency nowadays to use vibrators rectally, for added sensual stimulation. Indeed, some brands are actually *sold* as 'rectal vibrators' (they're a lot thinner than the ordinary kind).

Using rectal vibrators is absolute madness. Quite apart from the hygiene problem mentioned in earlier chapters, there's the all-important fact that a vibrator can disappear up your bottom, never to be seen again! Or – to be more precise – it *will* be seen again, after a surgeon has operated on you to remove it.

The less serious point is this. Before you buy a vibrator, you should appreciate that virtually all these devices are very noisy! If you live with your in-laws or in an apartment with thin walls, then most probably a vibrator is *not* for you.

into your love life. But in fact, nowadays you don't need to visit a shop to buy a 'vibe'.

In most liberated women's magazines, there are small ads indicating where you can purchase vibrators via mail order (or, perhaps one should say, female order . . .).

Q I am 25 years old and still a virgin. Personally, I would like to remain like this for quite a while, but people keep suggesting there's something wrong with me because I haven't had sex. What do you think?

A Old Delvin, him say: 'Good for you'! I dislike efforts to make people 'conform' sexually. I think there's far too much pressure put on women to lose their virginity these days, particularly by blokes who use lines like: 'You must be lesbian if you don't want to have intercourse.'

So hang on to your virginity if you want to. Obviously, you'll miss out on some fun, but I have to admit you'll miss out on a lot of monthly anxiety too.

Wife-swapping

Everything I've said about the dangers of open marriage applies with even more force to wife-swapping. This practice is now endemic in the relatively affluent suburbs of cities in the USA, Britain and Australia.

What usually happens is that a couple advertise in a 'contact magazine', and then selects a husband and wife from the replies they get – and I gather they get many.

They then meet up in a pub or bar, and see if they like the look of each other. If they do, they simply swap partners for the night.

The risks involved – particularly that of VD – are considerable. By going in for this kind of thing, you also put yourself in jeopardy of blackmail. A small number of couples who have indulged in it have been horrified to find their names splashed over the racier newspapers.

All of this makes it *very* dangerous living indeed (like 'feasting with panthers', as Oscar Wilde used to say in a different context).